Symposium in Immunology VI

Springer
Berlin
Heidelberg
New York
Barcelona
Budapest
Hong Kong
London
Milan
Paris
Santa Clara
Singapore
Tokyo

M. M. Eibl C. Huber
H. H. Peter U. Wahn (Eds.)

Symposium in Immunology VI

Tumor Immunology

With 27 Figures and 19 Tables

Springer

Prof. Dr. MARTHA M. EIBL
Institut für Immunologie der Universität Wien
Borschkegasse 8 a
1090 Wien
Austria

Prof Dr. CHRISTOPH HUBER
Department of Hematology
Johannes Gutenberg Universität
Langenbeckstr. 1
55101 Mainz
Germany

Prof. Dr. HANS H. PETER
Abteilung für Rheumatologie und
Klinische Immunologie
Medizinische Universitätsklinik
Hugstetter Str. 55
79106 Freiburg
Germany

Prof. Dr. ULRICH WAHN
Pädiatrische Pneumologie und Immunologie
Universitäts-Klinikum Rudolf-Virchow
Standort Charlottenburg
Heubnerweg 6
14059 Berlin
Germany

ISBN-13:978-3-540-61755-6 e-ISBN-13:978-3-642-60562-8
DOI: 10.1007/978-3-642-60562-8

Library of Congress Cataloging-in-Publication Data
Symposium in Immunology (5th : 1996 : Prague, Czech Republic) Symposium in Immunology VI : Tumor immunology / [edited by M. M. Eibl]. p. cm. ISBN-13:978-3-540-61755-6 (softcover : alk. paper)1. Tumor-Immunological-Congresses. I. Eibl, Martha M. II. Title. QR188.6.S96 1996 616.99'207'9-dc20 96-35941

Typesetting. Zechnersche Buchdruckerei, D-67346 Speyer
Cover design: Design & Production, D-69121 Heidelberg
Production: PRO EDIT GmbH, D-69126 Heidelberg
SPIN: 10543301 27/3136/ 543210 – Printed on acid-free paper

Contents

Therapeutic Approaches: Cytokines and Vaccines

Contributors

W. Aulitzky
Robert-Bosch-Krankenhaus, Zentrum für Innere Medizin
Department of Internal Medicine II
Auerbachstr. 110, D-70376 Stuttgart, Germany

D. Brändle
Ludwig Institute for Cancer Research, Brussels Branch, and
Cellular Genetics Unit of the Université Catholique de Louvain
74 Avenue Hippocrate, B-1200 Brussels, Belgium

V. Brichard
Ludwig Institute for Cancer Research, Brussels Branch, and
Cellular Genetics Unit of the Université Catholique de Louvain
74 Avenue Hippocrate, B-1200 Brussels, Belgium

T. Boon
Ludwig Institute for Cancer Research, Brussels Branch, and
Cellular Genetics Unit of the Université Catholique de Louvain
74 Avenue Hippocrate, B-1200 Brussels, Belgium

P. Coulie
Ludwig Institute for Cancer Research, Brussels Branch, and
Cellular Genetics Unit of the Université Catholique de Louvain
74 Avenue Hippocrate, B-1200 Brussels, Belgium

P. Fisch
Department of Medicine I (Hematology/Oncology),
Albert Ludwigs University
Hugstetter Straße 55, D-79106 Freiburg, Germany

G. Gaudernack
Section for Immunotherapy, Institute for Cancer Research
The Norwegian Radium Hospital
Montebello, N-0310 Oslo, Norway

B. Gaugler
Ludwig Institute for Cancer Research, Brussels Branch, and
Cellular Genetics Unit of the Université Catholique de Louvain
74 Avenue Hippocrate, B-1200 Brussels, Belgium

Y. Guilloux
Ludwig Institute for Cancer Research, Brussels Branch, and
Cellular Genetics Unit of the Université Catholique de Louvain
74 Avenue Hippocrate, B-1200 Brussels, Belgium

A. Habicht
Project Group Gene Therapy of Human Malignancies,
DKFZ – German Cancer Research Center
Im Neuenheimer Feld 280, D-69120 Heidelberg, Germany

M. Hauer
I. Medizinische Klinik und Poliklinik, Johannes Gutenberg University
Langenbeckstraße 1, D-55101 Mainz, Germany

B. Herbst
Department of Medicine I (Hematology/Oncology) and
Department of Biology, Albert Ludwigs University
Hugstetter Straße 55, D-79106 Freiburg, Germany

W. Herr
I. Medizinische Klinik und Poliklinik, Johannes Gutenberg University
Langenbeckstraße 1, D-55101 Mainz, Germany

C. Huber
Division of Haematology, Johannes Gutenberg University
Langenbeckstraße 1, D-55101 Mainz, Germany

E. Jäger
Department of Internal Medicine II,
Haematology – Oncology, Krankenhaus Nordwest
Steinbacher Hohl 2–26, D-60488 Frankfurt am Main, Germany

S. V. Kaveri
INSERM U430 and Université Pierre et Marie Curie, Hôpital Broussais
96, Rue Didot, F-75014 Paris, France

M. D. Kazatchkine
INSERM U430 and Université Pierre et Marie Curie, Hôpital Broussais
96, Rue Didot, F-75014 Paris, France

A. Knuth
Department of Internal Medicine II,
Haematology – Oncology, Krankenhaus Nordwest
Steinbacher Hohl 2–26, D-60488 Frankfurt, Germany

G. Köhler
Department of Pathology, Albert Ludwigs University
Albertstraße 19, D-79104 Freiburg, Germany

H. J. KOLB
Medizinische Klinik und Poliklinik III, Klinikum Großhadern
Ludwig Maximilians University
Marchioninistraße 15, D-81377 Munich, Germany

M. LINDAUER
Project Group Gene Therapy of Human Malignancies,
DKFZ – German Cancer Research Center
Im Neuenheimer Feld 280, D-69120 Heidelberg, Germany

A. LINDEMANN
Department of Medicine I (Hematology/Oncology)
Albert Ludwigs University
Hugstetter Straße 55, D-79106 Freiburg, Germany

J. LUSTGARTEN
The Scipps Research Institute, Immunology Department – IMM 15
10666 North Torrey Pines Road, La Jolla, CA 92037, USA

A. MACKENSEN
Department of Medicine I (Hematology/Oncology),
Albert Ludwigs University
Hugstetter Straße 55, D-79106 Freiburg, Germany

R. MERTELSMANN
Department of Medicine I (Hematology/Oncology),
Albert Ludwigs University
Hugstetter Straße 55, D-79106 Freiburg, Germany

S. MEUER
Institute of Immunology, Ruprecht Karls University
Im Neuenheimer Feld 305, D-69120 Heidelberg, Germany

U. MOEBIUS
Project Group Gene Therapy of Human Malignancies,
DKFZ – German Cancer Research Center
Im Neuenheimer Feld 280, D-69120 Heidelberg, Germany

M. PETER
Tumor Immunology Program, DKFZ – German Cancer Research Center
Im Neuenheimer Feld 280, D-69120 Heidelberg, Germany

A. PEZZUTTO
Robert-Rössle-Klinik, Virchow Klinikum
Humboldt University
Lindenberger Weg 80, D-13125 Berlin, Germany

F. M. Rosenthal
Department of Medicine I (Hematology/Oncology),
Albert Ludwigs University
Hugstetter Straße 55, D-79106 Freiburg, Germany

W. Rudy
Project Group Gene Therapy of Human Malignancies,
DKFZ – German Cancer Research Center
Im Neuenheimer Feld 280, D-69120 Heidelberg, Germany

J. Schneider
I. Medizinische Klinik und Poliklinik, Johannes Gutenberg University
Langenbeckstraße 1, D-55101 Mainz, Germany

B. Seliger
Department of Internal Medicine III, Division of Haematology/Oncology
Johannes Gutenberg University
Langenbeckstraße 1, D-55101 Mainz, Germany

L. A. Sherman
The Scripps Research Institute, Department of Immunology, IMM-15
10666 North Torrey Pines Road, La Jolla, CA 92037, USA

P. K. Srivastava
Department of Biological Sciences
Fordham University
300 Larkin Hall, Bronx, NY 10458, USA

M. Theobald
The Scripps Research Institute, Immunology Department – IMM 15
10666 North Torrey Pines Road, La Jolla, CA 92037, USA

P. van der Bruggen
Ludwig Institute for Cancer Research, Brussels Branch, and
Cellular Genetics Unit of the Université Catholique de Louvain
74 Avenue Hippocrate, B-1200 Brussels, Belgium

B. J. van den Eynde
Ludwig Institute for Cancer Research, Brussels Branch, and
Cellular Genetics Unit of the Université Catholique de Louvain
74 Avenue Hippocrate, B-1200 Brussels, Belgium

H. Veelken
Departmetn of Medicine I (Hematology/Oncology),
Albert Ludwigs University
Hugstetter Straße 55, D-79106 Freiburg, Germany

J. Westermann
Robert-Rössle-Klinik, Virchow Klinikum, Humboldt University
Lindenberger Weg 80, D-13125 Berlin, Germany

C. Wölfel
I. Medizinische Klinik und Poliklinik, Johannes Gutenberg University
Langenbeckstraße 1, D-55101 Mainz, Germany

T. Wölfel
I. Medizinische Klinik und Poliklinik
Johannes Gutenberg University
Langenbeckstraße 1, D-55101 Mainz, Germany

G. Wolff-Vorbeck
Department of Surgery, Albert Ludwigs University
Hugstetter Straße 55, D-79106 Freiburg, Germany

Characterization of Antigens Recognized by T Cells on Human Tumors

B. J. Van den Eynde, B. Gaugler, D. Brändle, Y. Guilloux, P. van der Bruggen, P. Coulie, V. Brichard, and T. Boon

Introduction

Tumor immunology has come into the limelight since the realization that antitumor cytotoxic T lymphocytes (CTLs), which constitute the major effectors involved in tumor rejection, can be cultured in vitro and used as tools to identify the target antigens expressed by the tumor cells (Boon et al. 1994). Tumor-specific CTLs have been found in most mouse tumor models, and in several human tumor types, mainly in melanoma. By using a genetic approach based on the transfection of genomic or cDNA libraries, we cloned the genes encoding a number of melanoma antigens. This led to the molecular identification of these antigens which usually consist of a peptide derived from an intracellular protein and presented to CTLs by an HLA class I molecule. On the basis of their pattern of expression, these antigens can be classified into three groups. Antigens of the first group are encoded by genes that are expressed in the tumor cells but are silent in normal adult tissues except the testis. The second group consists of differentiation antigens that are expressed in melanoma and in normal melanocytes. Antigens of the third group are unique to individual tumors and appear through tumor-specific mutations in genes expressed ubiquitously.

Tumor-Specific Antigens

Tumor-specific antigens are encoded by genes such as MAGE, BAGE or GAGE. Their specific expression in tumors and the fact that they are shared by a number of independent tumors make these antigens potentially useful for specific active immunotherapy of cancer. Remarkably, most CTLs directed against these antigens were derived from the same patient with metastatic melanoma whose outcome was extraordinarily favorable. Blood samples from other patients with a tumor expressing some or all of these genes were tested and no such CTLs were obtained by stimulating the lymphocytes with autologous tumor cells.

Symposium in Immunology VI
Eibl/Huber/Peter/Wahn (Eds.)

The MAGE Gene Family

The first antigen to be identified on human melanoma was antigen MZ2-E which is one of several antigens recognized by CTLs of patient MZ2 on the autologous melanoma cell line MZ2-MEL. A cosmid library was prepared with DNA from MZ2-MEL cells and transfected into an MZ2-MEL.E- antigen-negative variant together with a plasmid conferring resistance to geneticin. Transfectants expressing antigen MZ2-E were identified by their ability to stimulate the anti-E CTLs to release tumor necrosis factor (TNF; Traversari et al. 1992a). From such a transfectant, a cosmid was retrieved that transferred the expression of the antigen. This led to the identification of a new gene called MAGE-1 which codes for antigen MZ2-E (van der Bruggen et al. 1991).

Gene MAGE-1 is about 5 kb long and comprises two short exons and a long exon. An open reading frame coding for a protein of 309 amino acids is located in the third exon. The sequence of the MAGE-1 gene of melanoma cells is identical to that of a MAGE-1 gene isolated from normal blood cells of patient MZ2 (van der Bruggen et al. 1991). MAGE-1 is a member of a family of at least 12 closely related genes all located on chromosome X (De Plaen et al. 1994). The function of the MAGE proteins is unknown.

The expression of MAGE genes in various tumors and normal tissues was analyzed by reverse transcription and polymerase chain reaction amplification (RT-PCR) using primers specific for each MAGE gene. No expression of MAGE-1 was found in normal tissues, except in testis. Forty-eight percent of

Table 1. Expression of the genes MAGE-1, -3, BAGE, GAGE, and RAGE in tumor samples[a]

Histological type	Percentage of tumors positive for				
	MAGE-1	MAGE-3	BAGE	GAGE-1,2	RAGE-1
Melanomas					
Primary lesions	16	36	8	13	2
Metastases	48	76	26	28	5
Non-small cell lung carcinomas	49	47	4	19	0
Head and neck tumors	28	49	8	19	2
Bladder carcinomas	22	36	15	12	5
Sarcomas	14	24	6	25	14
Mammary carcinomas	18	11	10	9	1
Prostatic carcinomas	15	15	0	10	0
Colorectal carcinomas	2	17	0	0	0
Renal carcinomas	0	0	0	0	2
Leukemias and lymphomas	0	0	0	1	0
Testicular seminomas	4/6	3/6	1/6	5/6	0/3

[a] Expression was measured by RT-PCR on total RNA using primers specific for each gene.

metastatic melanoma samples were positive for MAGE-1 (Table 1) (Brasseur et al. 1995). Besides melanomas, a significant proportion of breast tumors (Brasseur et al. 1992), non-small cell lung carcinomas (Weynants et al. 1994), and head and neck carcinomas express MAGE-1 (Table 1).

Antigen MZ2-E consists of a nine-amino-acid peptide derived from the MAGE-1 protein and presented by HLA-A1 (Traversari et al. 1992b). Cell lines expressing MAGE-1 and HLA-A1 are recognized by the anti-MZ2-E CTL. About 26% of Caucasians express the HLA-A1 allele. Since 48% of metastatic melanomas express MAGE-1, about 12% of all metastatic melanomas are expected to express antigen MZ2-E.

Several other anti-tumor CTL clones of patient MZ2 were found to recognize another antigen which was named MZ2-Bb. The MZ2-Bb antigen was found to be presented by HLA-Cw16. When COS-7 cells were cotransfected with HLA-Cw16 and MAGE-1 cDNA, the transfectants stimulated the CTLs to produce TNF (van der Bruggen et al. 1994a). The MAGE-1.Cw16 antigenic peptide is a nonamer that is different from the MAGE-1.A1 peptide (Table 2). Thus, two different peptides derived from the MAGE-1 protein can bind to different HLA class I molecules within the same cells and constitute two antigens recognized by different CTLs.

Yet another anti-tumor CTL clone of patient MZ2 was analyzed. When tested on a panel of melanoma cell lines it was found to recognize tumors that expressed both HLA-A1 and MAGE-3 (Gaugler et al. 1994). Moreover, COS-7 cells cotransfected with HLA-A1 and MAGE-3 stimulated the CTLs. The MAGE-3.A1 antigenic peptide was identified as EVDPIGHLY (Table 2). The same peptide extended by one residue at its N-terminus is also presented to CTLs by HLA-B44 (Herman et al. 1996). Like MAGE-1, gene MAGE-3 is silent in normal tissues except testis, and is expressed in a number of tumors of different histological types (Table 1). Since MAGE-3 is more often expressed by melanomas than MAGE-1, it has a wider applicability for specific anti-tumor immunization of melanoma patients. Moreover, most of the MAGE-1-positive melanomas also express MAGE-3, which would allow the simultaneous immunization of these patients against both MAGE-1 and MAGE-3 antigens.

Another antigenic peptide derived from gene MAGE-3 was recently identified by a very different approach. Because the consensus motif for binding to HLA-A2 is well characterized and because HLA-A2 is the most frequent HLA class I allele (49% of Caucasians), we searched the MAGE-3 protein sequence for peptides that fitted the A2-binding motif. Nine such peptides were localized and synthesized. They were tested in vitro for their capacity to bind to HLA-A2 and the three best binders were used for in vitro stimulation of blood lymphocytes from normal HLA-A2 individuals. The responder cells were cloned and CTL clones were obtained that specifically lysed HLA-A2+ cells incubated with peptide FLWGPRALV (Table 2). These CTLs also recognized HLA-A2+melanoma cells expressing gene MAGE-3 (van der Bruggen et al. 1994b).

Table 2. Tumor-specific antigens shared by different tumors

Gene	Normal expression	MHC	Peptide	Position	Reference
MAGE-1	Testis	HLA-A1	EADPTGHSY	161–169	Traversari et al. 1992b
		HLA-Cw16	SAYGEPRKL	230–238	van der Bruggen et al. 1994a
MAGE-3	Testis	HLA-A1	EVDPIGHLY	168–176	Gaugler et al. 1994
		HLA-A2	FLWGPRALV	271–279	van der Bruggen et al. 1994b
		HLA-B44	MEVDPIGHLY	167–176	Herman et al. 1996
BAGE	Testis	HLA-Cw16	AARAVFLAL	2–10	Boël et al. 1995
GAGE-1/2	Testis	HLA-Cw6	YRPRPRRY	9–16	Van den Eynde et al. 1995
GAGE-3-6	Testis	HLA-A29	–	–	
RAGE-1	Retina	HLA-B7	–	–	
GnTV (atypical transcript)	None	HLA-A2	VLPDVFIRC	38–64	Guilloux et al. 1996

BAGE Gene

Another gene was identified by the genetic approach and found to encode an antigen recognized by autologous CTLs on MZ2-MEL cells. This new gene was named BAGE. It codes for a small protein of 43 amino acids that includes a peptide which is presented to CTLs by HLA-Cw16 (Table 2; Boël et al. 1995). Like the MAGE genes, BAGE is not expressed in normal tissues except testis, and is expressed in a number of tumors of various histologies (Table 1).

The GAGE Gene Family

Another family of genes, named GAGE, was recently identified by a similar approach using CTLs derived from the same melanoma patient (Van den Eynde et al. 1995). Six different cDNAs were identified, encoding proteins of 116–138 amino acids. GAGE-1 and GAGE-2 encode a peptide that is presented to CTLs by HLA-Cw6, whereas GAGE-3,-4,-5, and-6 encode a peptide which is presented by HLA-A29 (Table 2). Again, these genes are silent in normal adult tissues besides testis, but are expressed in a significant proportion of tumors of various types (Table 1).

RAGE Gene

Even though they are expressed on various types of tumors, all of these antigens were characterized on a single tumor type—melanoma. We recently used a similar approach to characterize antigens recognized by CTLs on a kidney tumor. We derived CTL clones directed against an antigen expressed on several renal cell carcinoma lines and presented by HLA-B7. This antigen was found to be encoded by a previously unknown gene that we called RAGE (Gaugler et al. 1996). This gene is silent in normal tissues except retina, and is expressed in a small proportion of tumors, mainly in sarcomas, bladder tumors and melanomas (Table 2). Since most retinal cells do not express major histocompatibility complex (MHC) class I molecules, this antigen is probably tumor-specific, although the formal proof of this will require the identification of the retinal cell type that expresses RAGE.

Antigen NA17-A

The recent characterization of antigen NA 17-A revealed that a very peculiar mechanism is responsible for the expression of this antigen on melanomas. Here it seems that a gene that is ubiquitously expressed, namely N-acetylglucosaminyltransferase V, contains an intron which itself appears to carry near its end a promoter that is activated only in melanoma cells (Guilloux et al. 1996). This atypical activation occurs in more than 50 % of melanomas. This produces a message containing a new open reading frame, which codes for the antigenic peptide in its intronic part. This peptide is presented by HLA-A2 to melanoma-specific CTLs (Table 2).

Differentiation Antigens

The observation that autologous CTLs can be generated readily against differentiation antigens present on normal melanocytes as well as melanoma cells was unexpected. Four genes encoding melanoma differentiation antigens have been identified: tyrosinase, Melan-A/Mart-1, gp100, and gp75 (Brichard et al. 1993; Bakker et al. 1994; Coulie et al. 1994; Cox et al. 1994; Kawakami et al. 1994a; Wang et al. 1995). Most of the identified antigenic peptides are presented by HLA-A2, but other HLA-peptide combinations have been found (Cox et al. 1994; Kawakami et al. 1994b; Kawakami et al. 1994c; Robbins et al. 1994; Topalian et al. 1994; Wölfel et al. 1994; Castelli et al. 1995; Kawakami et al. 1995; Wang et al. 1995; Brichard et al. 1996). One tyrosinase peptide is presented by HLA-DR4 to CD4 T cells (Topalian et al. 1994).

The pattern of CTL precursors directed against these differentiation antigens appears to be very different from that observed with the MAGE-like antigens. In effect, most melanoma patients have CTL precursors against differentiation antigens. These CTLs can be readily restimulated in vitro with autologous tumor cells and were found both in blood lymphocytes and in tumor-infiltrating lymphocytes (TIL) (Sensi et al. 1995; Brichard et al. 1996, Robbins et al. 1994). How these findings affect the immunotherapy potential of these antigens is unclear. The fact that many patients carry CTL precursors against these antigens implies that active immunization resulting in an increase in the number of these CTLs should be possible. On the other hand, the fact that many of these patients have progressive disease suggests that these CTLs are not very effective.

There is concern for the potential side effects of active or passive immunization against melanoma differentiation antigens. Not so much for the skin, where vitiligo due to the destruction of melanocytes might occur, but for the retina where melanocytes are present in the choroid layer. However, vitiligo has been associated with good prognoses in melanoma and also with adoptive transfer of TILs, without noticeable eye lesions (Bystryn et al. 1987; Richards et al 1992; Kawakami et al. 1994b; Kawakami et al. 1995). Carefully devised immunotherapy trials based on these antigens therefore seem reasonable.

Unique Antigens

Several years ago, the study of immunogenic variants of mouse tumors obtained by mutagenesis showed that point mutations in genes expressed ubiquitously could create antigenic epitopes recognized by CTLs (Boon 1992). Subsequent work on mouse tumors provided two interesting examples of tumor antigens resulting from point mutations (Mandelboim et al. 1994; Monach et al. 1995). This mechanism also accounts for the expression of antigens by human melanoma cells. As was seen with the mouse antigens induced by mutagens, the mutations are located in the region coding for the antigenic peptide, enabling it to bind to the MHC molecule or generating a new epitope. The first example is a point mutation in a previously unknown gene that produces a new antigenic peptide which, remarkably, is partially encoded by the 5' end of an intron (Coulie et al. 1995). Another example is a point mutation of the cyclin-dependent kinase 4 gene, which alters the regulation of the activity of this protein and may therefore contribute to oncogenesis (Wölfel et al. 1995). Point mutations may also create tumor antigens by directly altering an HLA molecule: we recently observed that autologous CTLs directed against a human renal cell carcinoma recognized an HLA-A2 molecule that was altered as a result of a point mutation changing one amino acid in the alpha-2 helix (Brändle et al. 1996).

It is expected that the antigens generated by point mutations are absolutely specific for the tumor cells, and that the CTL precursors directed against these antigens have not undergone any of the depletion or anergy that accompanies natural tolerance. However, these antigens are also expected to be unique for an individual tumor or restricted to very few tumors. This should make it difficult to develop therapeutic cancer vaccines based on these antigens. But one should not exclude the possibility that technological progress may one day make the identification of such antigens so easy that strictly individual immunogens will become a realistic possibility.

Clinical Prospects

Specific active immunotherapy as an adjuvant treatment of cancer has become a rational experimental approach since the molecular identification of tumor antigens recognized by CTLs. The most promising class of antigens are the shared tumor-specific antigens (Table 1). The expression of the MAGE, BAGE, and GAGE genes in the testis should not cause undesirable autoimmunity after immunization against such antigens. This was suggested by immunization studies of male mice against the tumor antigen encoded by the mouse gene P1A which is also expressed in testis. Despite a strong CTL response against this antigen, the immunized males were fertile and did not show any testicular inflammation (C. Uyttenhove, manuscript in preparation). This is probably because the testicular cells expressing the genes are germ cells which do not express MHC class I molecules and therefore do not constitute CTL targets (Haas et al. 1988; Takahashi et al. 1995).

The next few years will see the evaluation of new clinical trials using these defined tumor antigens. Progress at three different levels is anticipated. Firstly, a knowledge of the molecular nature of these antigens allows the selection of patients whose tumor actually expresses a given antigen. Eligible tumors should express the relevant gene along with the appropriate HLA class I specificity, and this can be tested readily by RT-PCR on RNA extracted from a small tumor sample. The fraction of tumors expressing a given antigen can be calculated from the frequency of expression of the relevant gene in that tumor type and from the frequency of the given class I molecule in the population. In Caucasians, about 60 % of melanomas express at least one of the tumor-specific antigens thus far defined.

Secondly, the definition of the molecular nature of tumor antigens allows the rational design of highly specific vaccine preparations. These could consist of engineered cells expressing the antigens or of antigenic peptides mixed with appropriate adjuvants. The availability of the genes encoding the antigens also allows the preparation of recombinant proteins that can be combined with adjuvants, or the preparation of recombinant viral vectors that can be used for immunization .

Thirdly, the precise knowledge of the antigenic epitopes involved in the immune response of an individual patient against his own tumor cells allows a careful monitoring of the CTL responses to these epitopes after the vaccination. This should help to optimize the immunization procedure.

It is impossible now to predict the clinical outcome of such strategies, but preliminary results with the MAGE-3.A1 peptide are promising (Marchand et al. 1995). Since a number of tumors appear to express several antigens, patients bearing these tumors could be immunized simultaneously with several distinct and defined antigens. This should eliminate the tumor cells more effectively. It should also reduce the emergence of antigen-negative variants arising by the loss of antigen expression, as it is unlikely that the same variant would simultaneously loose distinct nominal antigens.

References

Bakker ABH, Schreurs MWJ, de Boer AJ, Kawakami Y, Rosenberg SA, Adema GJ, Figdor CG (1994) Melanocyte lineage-specific antigen gp100 is recognized by melanoma-derived tumor-infiltrating lymphocytes. J Exp Med 179:1005–1009

Boël P, Wildmann C, Sensi M-L, Brasseur R, Renauld J-C, Coulie P, Boon T, van der Bruggen P (1995) BAGE, a new gene encoding an antigen recognized on human melanomas by cytolytic T lymphocytes. Immunity 2:167–175

Boon T (1992) Toward a Genetic Analysis of Tumor Rejection Antigens. Adv Cancer Res 58:177–210

Boon T, Cerottini J-C, Van den Eynde B, van der Bruggen P, Van Pel A (1994) Tumor antigens recognized by T lymphocytes. Annu Rev Immunol 12:337–365
Brändle D, Brasseur F, Weynants P, Boon T, Van den Eynde B (1996) A mutated HLA-A2 molecule recognized by autologous cytotoxic T lymphocytes on a human renal cell carcinoma. J Exp Med 183:2501–2508
Brasseur F, Marchand M, Vanwijck R, Hérin M, Lethé B, Chomez P, Boon T (1992) Human gene MAGE-1, which codes for a tumor rejection antigen, is expressed by some breast tumors. Int J Cancer 52:839–841
Brasseur F, Rimoldi D, Liénard D, Lethé B, Carrel S, Arienti F, Suter L, Vanwijck R, Bourlond A, Humblet Y, Vacca A, Conese M, Lahaye T, Degiovanni G, Deraemaecker R, Beauduin M, Sastre X, Salamon E, Dréno B, Jäger E, Knuth A, Chevreau C, Suciu S, Lachapelle M, Pouillart P, Parmiani G, Lejeune F, Cerottini J-C, Boon T, Marchand M (1995) Expression of MAGE genes in primary and metastatic cutaneous melanoma. Int J Cancer 63:375–380
Brichard V, Van Pel A, Wölfel T, Wölfel C, De Plaen E, Lethé B, Coulie P, Boon T (1993) The tyrosinase gene codes for an antigen recognized by autologous cytolytic T lymphocytes on HLA-A2 melanomas. J Exp Med 178:489–495
Brichard VG, Herman J, Van Pel A, Wildmann C, Gaugler B, Wölfel T, Boon T, Lethé B (1996) A tyrosinase nonapeptide presented by HLA-B44 is recognized on a human melanoma by autologous cytolytic T lymphocytes. Eur J Immunol 26:224–230
Bystryn J-C, Darrell R, Friedman RJ, Kopf A (1987) Prognostic significance of hypopigmentation in malignant melanoma. Arch Dermatol 123:1053–1055
Castelli C, Storkus WJ, Maeurer MJ, Martin DM, Huang EC, Pramanik BN, Nagabhushan TL, Parmiani G, Lotze MT (1995) Mass spectrometric identification of a naturally processed melanoma peptide recognized by CD8+ cytotoxic T lymphocytes. J Exp Med 181:363–368
Coulie PG, Brichard V, Van Pel A, Wölfel T, Schneider J, Traversari C, Mattei S, De Plaen E, Lurquin C, Szikora J-P, Renauld J-C, Boon T (1994) A new gene coding for a differentiation antigen recognized by autologous cytolytic T lymphocytes on HLA-A2 melanomas. J Exp Med 180:35–42
Coulie PG, Lehmann F, Lethé B, Herman J, Lurquin C, Andrawiss M, Boon T (1995) A mutated intron sequence codes for an antigenic peptide recognized by cytolytic T lymphocytes on a human melanoma. Proc Natl Acad Sci USA 92:7976–7980
Cox AL, Skipper J, Chen Y, Henderson RA, Darrow TL, Shabanowitz J, Engelhard VH, Hunt DF, Slingluff CL, Jr (1994) Identification of a peptide recognized by five melanoma-specific human cytotoxic T cell lines. Science 264:716–719
De Plaen E, Arden K, Traversari C, Gaforio JJ, Szikora J-P, De Smet C, Brasseur F, van der Bruggen P, Lethé B, Lurquin C, Brasseur R, Chomez P, De Backer O, Cavenee W, Boon T (1994) Structure, chromosomal localization and expression of twelve genes of the MAGE family. Immunogenetics 40:360–369
Gaugler B, Van den Eynde B, van der Bruggen P, Romero P, Gaforio JJ, De Plaen E, Lethé B, Brasseur F, Boon T (1994) Human gene MAGE-3 codes for an antigen recognized on a melanoma by autologous cytolytic T lymphocytes. J Exp Med 179:921–930
Gaugler B, Brouwenstijn N, Vantomme V, Szikora J-P, Van der Spek CW, Patard JJ, Boon T, Schrier P, Van den Eynde BJ (1996) A new gene coding for an antigen recognized by autologous CTL on a human renal carcinoma. Immunogenetics 44:323–330
Guilloux Y, Lucas S, Brichard VG, Van Pel A, Viret C, De Plaen E, Brasseur F, Lethé B, Jotereau F, Boon T (1996) A peptide recognized by human cytolytic T lymphocytes on HLA-A2 melanomas is encoded by an intron sequence of the N-acetylglucosaminyltransferase V gene. J Exp Med 183:1173–1183

Haas GG Jr, D'Cruz OJ, De Bault LE (1988)Distribution of human leukocyte antigen-ABC and -D/DR antigens in the unfixed human testis. Am J Reprod Immunol Microbiol 18:47–51

Herman J, van der Bruggen P, Luescher I, Mandruzzato S, Romero P, Thonnard J, Fleischhauer K, Boon T, Coulie PG (1996) A peptide encoded by human gene MAGE-3 and presented by HLA-B44 induces cytolytic T lymphocytes that recognize tumor cells expressing MAGE-3. Immunogenetics 43:377–383

Kawakami Y, Eliyahu S, Delgado CH, Robbins PF, Rivoltini L, Topalian SL, Miki T, Rosenberg SA (1994a) Cloning of the gene coding for a shared human melanoma antigen recognized by autologous T cells infiltrating into tumor. Proc Natl Acad Sci USA 91:3515–3519

Kawakami Y, Eliyahu S, Delgado CH, Robbins PF, Sakaguchi K, Appella E, Yannelli JR, Adema GJ, Miki T, Rosenberg SA (1994b) Identification of a human melanoma antigen recognized by tumor-infiltrating lymphocytes associated with in vivo tumor rejection. Proc Natl Acad Sci USA 91:6458–6462

Kawakami Y, Eliyahu S, Sakaguchi K, Robbins PF, Rivoltini L, Yannelli JR, Appella E, Rosenberg SA (1994c) Identification of the immunodominant peptides of the MART- 1 human melanoma antigen recognized by the majority of HLA-A2-restricted tumor infiltrating lymphocytes. J Exp Med 180:347–352

Kawakami Y, Eliyahu S, Jennings C, Sakaguchi K, Kang X, Southwood S, Robbins PF, Sette A, Appella E, Rosenberg SA (1995). Recognition of multiple epitopes in the human melanoma antigen gp100 by tumor-infiltrating T lymphocytes associated with in vivo tumor regression. J Immunol 154:3961–3968

Mandelboim O, Berke G, Fridkin M, Feldman M, Eisenstein M, Eisenbach L (1994) CTL induction by a tumour-associated antigen octapeptide derived from a murine lung carcinoma. Nature 369: 67–71

Marchand M, Weynants P, Rankin E, Arienti F, Belli F, Parmiani G, Cascinelli N, Bourlond A, Vanwijck R, Humblet Y, Canon J-L, Laurent C, Naeyaert J-M, Plagne R, Deraemaeker R, Knuth A, Jäger E, Brasseu F, Herman J, Coulie PG, Boon T (1995) Tumor regression responses in melanoma patients treated with a peptide encoded by gene MAGE-3. Int J Cancer 63:883–885

Monach PA, Meredith SC, Siegel CT, Schreiber H (1995) A unique tumor antigen produced by a single amino acid substitution. Immunity 2:45–59

Richards JM, Mehta N, Ramming K, Skosey P (1992) Sequential chemoimmunotherapy in the treatment of metastatic melanoma. J Clin Oncol 10:1338–1343

Robbins PF, El-Gamil, M, Kawakami Y, Rosenberg SA (1994) Recognition of tyrosinase by tumor-infiltrating lymphocytes from a patient responding to immunotherapy. Cancer Res 54:3124–3126

Sensi ML, Traversari C, Radrizzani M, Salvi S, Maccalli C, Mortarini R, Rivoltini L, Farina C, Nicolini G, Wölfel T, Brichard V, Boon T, Bordignon C, Anichini A, Parmiani G (1995) Cytotoxic T-lymphocyte clones from different patients display limited T-cell-receptor variable-region gene usage in HLA-A2-restricted recognition of the melanoma antigen Melan-A/MART-1. Proc Natl Acad Sci USA 92:5674–5678

Takahashi K, Shichijo S, Noguchi M, Hirohata M, Itoh K (1995) Identification of MAGE-1 and MAGE-4 proteins in spermatogonia and primary spermatocytes of testis. Cancer Res 55:3478–3482

Topalian SL, Rivoltini L, Mancini M, Markus NR, Robbins PF, Kawakami Y, Rosenberg SA (1994) Human CD4+ T cells specifically recognize a shared melanoma-associated antigen encoded by the tyrosinase gene. Proc Natl Acad Sci USA 91:9461–9465

Traversari C, van der Bruggen P, Van den Eynde B, Hainaut P, Lemoine C, Ohta N, Old L, Boon T (1992a) Transfection and expression of a gene coding for a human melanoma antigen recognized by autologous cytolytic T lymphocytes. Immunogenetics 35:145–152

Traversari C, van der Bruggen P, Luescher IF, Lurquin C, Chomez P, Van Pel A, De Plaen E, Amar-Costesec A, Boon T (1992b) A nonapeptide encoded by human gene MAGE-1 is recognized on HLA-A1 by cytolytic T lymphocytes directed against tumor antigen MZ2-E. J Exp Med 176:1453–1457

Van den Eynde B, Peeters O, De Backer O, Gaugler B, Lucas S, Boon T (1995). A new family of genes coding for an antigen recognized by autologous cytolytic T lymphocytes on a human melanoma. J Exp Med 182:689–698

van der Bruggen P, Traversari C, Chomez P, Lurquin C, De Plaen E, Van den Eynde B, Knuth A, Boon T (1991) A gene encoding an antigen recognized by cytolytic T lymphocytes on a human melanoma. Science 254:1643–1647

van der Bruggen P, Szikora J-P, Boël P, Wildmann C, Somville M, Sensi M, Boon T (1994a) Autologous cytolytic T lymphocytes recognize a MAGE-1 nonapeptide on melanomas expressing HLA-Cw*1601. Eur J Immunol 24:2134–2140

van der Bruggen P, Bastin J, Gajewski T, Coulie PG, Boël P, De Smet C, Traversari C, Townsend A, Boon T (1994b) A peptide encoded by human gene MAGE-3 and presented by HLA-A2 induces cytolytic T lymphocytes that recognize tumor cells expressing MAGE-3. Eur J Immunol 24:3038–3043

Wang R-F, Robbins PF, Kawakami Y, Kang X-Q, Rosenberg SA (1995). Identification of a gene encoding a melanoma tumor antigen recognized by HLA-A31-restricted tumor-infiltrating lymphocytes. J Exp Med 181:799–804

Weynants P, Lethé B, Brasseur F, Marchand M, Boon T (1994) Expression of MAGE genes by non-small cell lung carcinomas. Int J Cancer 56:826–829

Wölfel T, Van Pel A, Brichard V, Schneider J, Seliger B, Meyer zum Büschenfelde K-H, Boon T (1994) Two tyrosinase nonapeptides recognized on HLA-A2 melanomas by autologous cytolytic T lymphocytes. Eur J Immunol 24:759–764

Wölfel T, Hauer M, Schneider J, Serrano M, Wölfel C, Klehmann-Hieb E, De Plaen E, Hankeln T, Meyer zum Büschenfelde K-H, Beach D (1995) A $p16^{INK4a}$-insensitive CDK4 mutant targeted by cytolytic T lymphocytes in a human melanoma. Science 269:1281–1284

Shared and Individual CTL-Defined Antigens on Human Melanoma Cells

T. WÖLFEL, J. SCHNEIDER, M. HAUER, C. WÖLFEL, AND W. HERR

Cytolytic T lymphocytes (CTL) have been shown to mediate immune protection and rejection responses in animal tumor models. T lymphocytes recognize not intact proteins, but protein-derived peptides presented by HLA molecules on the cell surface. HLA-associated peptides originate from proteins of any cellular location. This allows T cells to survey the organism for any alteration occurring intracellularly and opens up an enormous variety of potential target antigens. For these reasons T-cell-defined antigens are considered as promising candidates for targeted immunotherapy.

Specificity of CTL Recognizing Autologous Melanoma Cells in Patient SK29(AV)

During the last 4 years we have concentrated on the identification of antigens recognized by melanoma-reactive T lymphocytes in patient SK29(AV), thereby continuing earlier work in this model (Livingston et al. 1979; Knuth et al. 1984, 1989; Wölfel et al. 1989). A panel of CTL clones was derived from responder lymphocytes of autologous mixed lymphocyte-tumor cell cultures (MLTCs). They lysed autologous melanoma cells, but not EBV-transformed B lymphocytes, and were predominantly restricted by HLA-A2.1. CTL not restricted by HLA-A2.1 were only found when variant melanoma cells lacking expression of HLA-A2.1 had been used as stimulators in MLTCs. According to immunoselection and antibody blocking experiments, the various CTL clones recognized at least four distinct antigens, named Aa, Ab, B, and C (Wölfel et al. 1993). This was confirmed by the observation that different CTL clones recognized peptides in distinct HPLC fractions containing naturally processed peptides eluted from HLA-A2.1 of SK29 melanoma cells (Wölfel et al. 1994a). While CTL against antigens SK29-Aa and -Ab lysed a high proportion of allogenic HLA-A2 melanoma lines, CTL against antigens SK29-B and -C apparently only lysed autologous melanoma cells (Wölfel et al. 1993) (see Fig. 1 for some CTL clones). Ab- and Aa-reactive CTL were also isolated from the blood of other patients (Wölfel et al. 1993; Coulie et al. 1994).

Symposium in Immunology VI
Eibl/Huber/Peter/Wahn (Eds.)

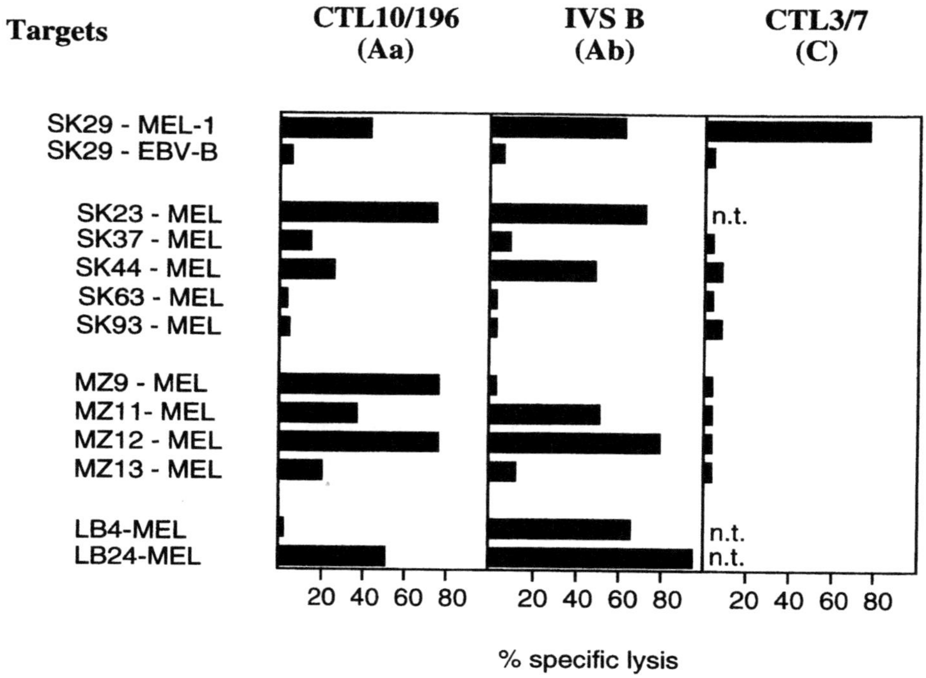

Fig. 1. Cross-reactivity of SK-29-CTL clones with allogeneic HLA-A2.1-positive melanoma lines. Data of a 4h-^{51}Cr release assay are given. CTL were added at a 30:1 effector to target cell ratio. Antigen specificities of CTL clones are noted in parentheses. **n.t.,** Not tested

Identification of Antigens SK29-Aa and -Ab as Melanocyte Differentiation Antigens

Together with Thierry Boon and his colleagues at the Ludwig Institute for Cancer Research in Brussels, we set out to identify shared melanoma antigens Aa and Ab using cDNA expression via COS cell transfection. This technique was initially applied to the cloning of cDNA encoding antibody-defined cell surface molecules (Seed and Aruffo 1987) and was later proposed for the cloning of T-cell epitopes (Karttunen et al. 1992). A cDNA library was prepared from SK29 melanoma cells and cDNA pools were cotransfected with the HLA-A2.1 gene in monkey kidney cells (COS-7). Antigen-expressing transfectants were detected according to their ability to induce tumor necrosis factor (TNF) production by CTL specific for Aa and Ab, respectively (Traversari et al. 1992). Positive cDNA pools were subcloned and cDNA clones were transfected again. Finally cDNA clones were identified that code for antigens Ab (Brichard et al. 1993) and Aa (Coulie et al. 1994).

The cDNA clone inducing recognition by Ab-specific CTL codes for tyrosinase (Brichard et al. 1993). Tyrosinase catalyzes the synthesis of the melanin precursor molecule dihydroxyphenylalanine (DOPA). It is not related to tyrosine hydroxylase, which also produces DOPA in adrenal cells and adrenergic neurons. HLA-A2.1-restricted tyrosinase-reactive CTL from the blood of two patients [SK29 (AV) and LB24] reacted with distinct epitopes (Wölfel et al. 1994b). SK29-CTL recognized peptide YMNGTMSQV (residues 368–376), whereas LB24-CTL recognized peptide MLLAVLYCL (residues 1–9). In peptide recognition assays both peptides had to be applied at significantly higher concentrations than previously published viral peptides also presented by HLA-A2.1. Even when targets were pretreated with monoclonal antibody MA2.1 to enhance binding of exogenous peptides (Bodmer et al. 1989), the concentrations of MLLAVLYCL and YMNGTMSQV required to give half-maximal lysis were around 0.1–1 μM. While for MLLAVLYCL this could be explained by its rather low binding affinity to HLA-A2.1, peptide YMNGTMSQV bound to HLA-A2 with an affinity comparable to known strongly binding viral peptide antigens. Recently, an explanation was found for its low target sensitizing ability. The naturally processed tyrosinase peptide 368–376 was purified from HLA-A2.1 molecules of melanoma cells and its sequence was determined as YMDGTMSQV with tandem mass spectrometry (Cox et al. 1994). It carried aspartic acid (D) instead of asparagine (N) at amino acid position 3. Peptide YMDGTMSQV was recognized by SK29-CTL in approximately 1000-fold lower concentrations than its genetically encoded counterpart. The modification occurring in this peptide resulted from enzymatic deamidation of residue 370. The possibility of posttranslational modification has an impact on the prediction of potential peptide antigens (Skipper et al. 1996).

Identical cDNA clones encoding antigen Aa were isolated in independent experiments with CTL of two melanoma patients [SK29(AV) and LB33] from the same cDNA library as tyrosinase cDNA (Coulie et al. 1994). It was named Melan-A and turned out to be identical to shared melanoma antigen MART-1 (Kawakami et al. 1994a). The function of the Melan-A/MART-1 protein is still unknown. All Melan-A/MART-1-reactive CTL derived from the blood of patient SK29(AV), which were restricted by HLA-A2.1, recognized the same peptide, EAAGIGILTV. This contains the immunodominant epitope targeted by a large proportion of HLA-A2.1-restricted melanoma-reactive T lymphocytes derived from different patients (Kawakami et al. 1994b). Moreover, from the same protein region a peptide is processed that is recognized by some SK29-CTL in association with HLA-B45.1. Its peptide sequence largely overlaps with the peptide presented by HLA-A2.1 (T. Wölfel, J. Schneider, unpublished data).

The sequences of cDNAs cloned from melanoma cells that encode melanocyte differentiation antigens tyrosinase and Melan-A/MART-1 are not altered. Among normal cells they are exclusively expressed in melanocytes. According to polymerase chain reaction (PCR) testing, approximately

50%–70% of melanoma cell lines express these antigens, while almost all melanoma tissues are positive (Coulie et al. 1994). These antigens represent normal autoantigens.

T cells recognizing melanocyte-associated differentiation antigens, such as tyrosinase and Melan-A/MART-1, have also been detected in the blood of normal donors (Visseren et al. 1995; Bakker et al. 1995; Herr et al. 1996). It is presently a matter of debate whether a relevant and profitable antimelanocyte immunity can be generated in melanoma patients (Nanda and Sercarz 1995) (see below).

Identification of Antigen SK29-C as Mutated Cyclin-Dependent Kinase 4

As mentioned above and demonstrated in Fig. 1, HLA-A2.1-restricted CTL against antigen SK29-C only lysed autologous tumor cells, but did not recognize autologous EBV-transformed B lymphocytes or a panel of allogeneic HLA-A2-positive melanoma cell lines. Using the COS transfection technique as for antigens Aa and Ab, we cloned cDNA for antigen SK29-C (Wölfel et al. 1995). Its sequence encodes cyclin-dependent kinase 4 (CDK4). When compared with homologous cDNA from normal cells, CDK4 cDNA of melanoma cells and melanoma tissue of patient SK29(AV) carries a C→T transition at the first nucleotide position of codon 24. This causes an arginine (R) to cystein (C) exchange at protein level, for which reason the mutant CDK4 was named CDK4-R24C. The R24C mutation resulted from a UV-typical C→T transition at a dipyrimidine site (Brash et al. 1991) probably occurring early in tumorigenesis. In vitro artefacts due to long-term cell culture as well as sequence alterations resulting from reverse transcription in the course of cDNA library construction were excluded as well as natural CDK4 polymorphism involving residue 24.

Cysteine 24 is part of the antigenic peptide CDK4-R24C peptide ACDPHSGHFV (amino acids 23–32). The mutated residue does not constitute the CTL epitope, but rather improves binding to HLA-A2.1. It is unclear whether the R24C mutation also influences peptide processing and transport or, in other words, whether the wild-type homologue of CDK4 peptide 23–32 appears on the cell surface at all.

Aside from its role in immune recognition, the R24C mutation also prevents binding of the CDK4 inhibitors $p16^{INK4a}$ and $p15^{INK4b}$, while the function of other CDK4 inhibitors is not impaired (Wölfel et al. 1995). Deregulated CDK4/cyclin D complexes, however, may acquire oncogenic potential. Therefore, it seems plausible to assume that expression of the CDK4-R24C allele contributed to the malignant phenotype in the SK29 melanoma. This view is supported by the frequent functional inactivation of $p16^{INK4a}$ in certain tumor types including melanoma (Kamb et al. 1994; Caldas et al. 1994;

Mori et al. 1994). In patient SK29(AV) the CDK4-R24 allele was generated by a somatic mutation. Recently, the same allele was found to be associated with the prevalence of melanoma in two families with hereditary melanoma. Among the members of both kindreds 11/11 melanoma patients carried the mutated allele, whereas only 2/24 unaffected individuals were carriers. The latter persons were younger than the mean age of melanoma occurrence in these families. The authors concluded that CDK4-R24C encodes a dominant oncogene (Zuo et al. 1996).

In addition to impairment of p16 inhibition, the mutated site of CDK4-R24C generates a tumor-specific target antigen for autologous CTL. Antigens with such dual functions were described as targets of potent tumor rejection responses in vivo in virally induced murine tumor models (Kast et al. 1989; Feltkamp et al. 1993). Whether CDK4-R24C constitutes a target for a rejection response in vivo remains to be proven. Notably, the patient survived metastatic disease and has been free of detectable tumor since 1978 (Livingston et al. 1979). Aside from the SK29 melanoma, we found the CDK4-R24C allele in 3 of 60 melanomas analyzed so far (C. Wölfel, U. Siepmann, T. Wölfel; unpublished data). The identification of a patient subgroup whose tumors carry the CDK4-R24C-allele will eventually allow study of whether the simultaneous expression of HLA-A2.1 and CDK4-R24C is associated with a more favorable clinical course, i.e., prolonged survival and/or improved response to immunotherapy.

Relevance of T-Cell-Defined Antigens in vivo and Implications for Therapeutic Vaccination

In the SK29 melanoma normal differentiation antigens and a mutated neoantigen constitute targets of autologous T lymphocytes (summarized in Fig. 2). Multiple antigens simultaneously present on tumor cells have also been described in other melanomas (Van den Eynde et al. 1989; Lehmann et al. 1995). Some of them have been characterized and are mostly structurally normal, like the proteins encoded by the MAGE, BAGE, and GAGE genes (see also B. Van den Eynde in this issue). Aside from CDK4-R24C, two further mutated CTL epitopes have been reported during the last year. These were MUM-1 (Coulie et al. 1995) and β-catenin-S37F (Robbins et al. 1996).

The identification of a variety of melanoma antigens already prompted the assumption that the majority of tumors carry antigens which are recognizable by autologous T lymphocytes (Prehn 1993). It is noteworthy that all known CTL-defined antigens were identified on progressive tumors, which at first sight might lead to the conclusion that they are irrelevant in vivo. However, the presence of T cell target antigens and clinical tumor progression are not mutually exclusive and can be explained with current observations or hypotheses on the induction of immune tolerance or ignorance:

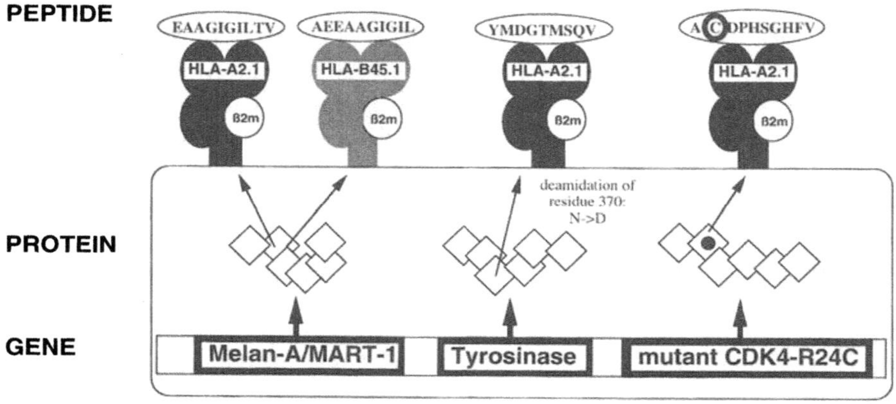

Fig. 2 Diagram of antigens recognized by autologous CTL clones on melanoma cells of patient SK29 (AV). ●, point mutation

- If antigen-presenting cells lack expression of costimulatory molecules (Becker et al. 1993) and hypothetical "danger signals" (Matzinger 1994), no protective immune response can be induced, but antigen-specific T cells become anergic instead.
- Observations in mouse models suggest that immune responses induced by weakly immunogenic tumors do not lead to rejection, but rather improve tumor growth. This phenomenon has been termed "tumor immunostimulation" (Prehn 1993).
- Tumors produce immunosuppressive cytokines, such as IL-10 and TGF-β (Luscher et al. 1994).

In animal experiments, vaccination of syngeneic animals with tumors led to protection against the immunizing tumor, but not to cross-protection against other syngenic tumors (Basombrio 1970; Srivastava and Old 1988). A recent report stated that vaccination with independently induced tumors sharing an antigen, which is known to efficiently induce CTL responses, did not lead to cross-protection (Ramarathinam et al. 1995). Certainly, systematic animal studies thoroughly addressing this issue would require immunization with known shared antigens using various vaccine strategies in different models. However, according to published mouse experiments, only individually distinct, not shared antigens elicit protective immunity. Individual antigens have been identified in a few human tumors (see above). Although it is unclear whether they can induce rejection responses in vivo, their existence justifies the use of autologous tumor tissues as a source for vaccine preparations such as autologous tumor cells, i.e., modified by viruses (Schirrmacher 1992) or gene transfer (Colombo and Forni 1994), autologous peptide-loaded heat shock proteins (Srivastava et al. 1994)(see chapter by Srivastava, this volume) or unfractionated peptide pools eluted from tumor tissues (Zitvogel et al. 1996). A common pitfall is that the antigens contained in these preparations are unknown. If such immunization trials fail it will be impossible to distinguish between lack of antigenicity and inappropriate vaccination.

With respect to T-cell-based immunotherapy with defined antigens in human cancer, at present shared antigenic epitopes are the only ones to be applicable in a significant proportion of patients. Moreover both in mice and in humans, immune responses to normal autoantigens also expressed on tumors have been associated with improved survival (Hara et al. 1995; Bystryn et al. 1987). Indeed, vaccination trials applying MAGE peptides and peptides of melanocyte differentiation antigens have been initiated with encouraging first results as reported in this volume (see chapters by Van den Eynde and Knuth). If this initial success is confirmed in a larger number of patients with advanced disease, patients in earlier disease stages, who are at high risk of relapse or metastatic spread, will be included in these trials. The aim of therapeutic immunizations will be to complement conventional therapies such as surgery or chemotherapy in patients whose tumors have not yet lost their antigenicity. Major areas of interest for the next few years are

- the search for new antigens that have ideal characteristics, such as tumor-restricted expression, stable expression, occurrence in a significant proportion of individual tumors and presentation by frequent HLA alleles;
- the development of vaccine adjuvants and delivery systems.

References

Bakker AB, Marland G, de Boer A, Huijbens RJ, Danen EH, Adema GJ, Figdor CG (1995) Generation of antimelanoma cytotoxic T lymphocytes from healthy donors after presentation of melanoma-associated antigen-derived epitopes by dendritic cells in vitro. Cancer Res 55:5330–5334

Basombrio MA (1970) Search for common antigenicities among twenty-five sarcomas induced by methylcholanthrene. Cancer Res 30:2458–2462

Becker JC, Brabletz T, Czerny C, Termeer C, Brocker EB (1983) Tumor escape mechanisms from immunosurveillance: induction of unresponsiveness in a specific MHC-restricted CD4+ human T cell clone by the autologous MHC class II+ melanoma. Int Immunol 5:1501–1508

Bodmer H, Ogg G, Gotch F, McMichael A (1989) Anti-HLA-A2 antibody-enhancement of peptide association with HLA-A2 as detected by cytotoxic T lymphocytes. Nature 342:443–446

Brash DE, Rudolph JA, Simon JA, Lin A, McKenna GJ, Baden HP, Halperin AJ, Ponten J (1991) A role for sunlight in skin cancer: UV-induced p53 mutations in squamous cell carcinoma. Proc Natl Acad Sci USA 88:10124–10128

Brichard V, Van Pel A, Wölfel T, Wölfel C, De Plaen E, Lethé B, Coulie P, Boon T (1993) The tyrosinase gene codes for an antigen recognized by autologous cytolytic T lymphocytes on HLA-A2 melanomas. J Exp Med 178:489–495

Bystryn J-C, Darrell R, Friedman RJ, Kopf A (1987) Prognostic significance of hypopigmentation in malignant melanoma. Arch Dermatol 123:1053–1055

Caldas C, Hahn SA, da Costa LT, Redston MS, Schutte M, Seymour AB, Weinstein CL, Hruban RH, Yeo CJ, Kern SE (1994) Frequent somatic mutations and homozygous deletions of the p16 (MTS1) gene in pancreatic adenocarcinoma [published erratum appears in Nat Genet 1994 Dec; 8(4):410]. Nat Genet 8:27–32

Colombo MP, Forni G (1994) Cytokine gene transfer in tumor inhibition and tumor therapy. Immunol today 15:48–51

Coulie P, Brichard V, Van Pel A, Wölfel T, Schneider J, Traversari C, Mattei S, De Plaen E, Lurquin C, Szikora J-P, Renauld J-C, Boon T (1994) A new gene coding for a differentiation antigen recognized by autologous cytolytic T lymphocytes on HLA-A2 melanomas. J Exp Med 180:35–42

Coulie PG, Lehmann F, Lethé B, Herman J, Lurquin C, Andrawiss M, Boon T (1995) A mutated intron sequence codes for an antigenic peptide recognized by cytolytic T lymphocytes on a human melanoma. Proc Natl Acad Sci USA 92:7976–7980

Cox AL, Skipper J, Chen Y, Henderson RA, Darrow TL, Shabanowitz J, Engelhard VH, Hunt DF, Slingluff Jr. CL (1994) Identification of a peptide recognized by five melanoma-specific human cytotoxic T cell lines. Science 264:716–719

Feltkamp MC, Smits HL, Vierboom MP, Minnaar RP, de Jongh BM, Drijfhout JW, ter Schegget J, Melief CJ, Kast WM (1993) Vaccination with cytotoxic T lymphocyte epitope-containing peptide protects against a tumor induced by human papillomavirus type 16-transformed cells. Eur J Immunol 23:2242–2249

Hara I, Takechi Y, Houghton AN (1995) Implicating a role for immune recognition of self in tumor rejection: passive immunization against the Brown locus protein. J Exp Med 182:1609–1614

Herr W, Schneider J, Lohse AW, Meyer zum Büschenfelde K-H, Wölfel T (1996) Detection and quantification of blood-derived CD8+ T lymphocytes secreting tumor necrosis factor alpha in response to HLA-A2.1-binding melanoma and viral peptide antigens. J Immunol Method 191:131–142

Kamb A, Gruis NA, Weaver-Feldhaus J, Liu Q, Harshman K, Tavtigian SV, Stockert E, Day III RS, Johnson BE, Skolnick MH (1994) A cell cycle regulator potentially involved in genesis of many tumor types. Science 264:436–440

Karttunen J, Sanderson S, Shastri N (1992) Detection of rare antigen-presenting cells by the lacZ T-cell activation assay suggests an expression cloning strategy for T-cell antigens. Proc Natl Acad Sci USA 89:6020–6024

Kast WM, Offringa R, Peters PJ, Voordouw AC, Meloen RH, van der Eb AJ, Melief CJM (1989) Eradication of adenovirus E1-induced tumors by E1A-specific cytotoxic lymphocytes. Cell 59:603–614

Kawakami Y, Eliyahu S, Delgado CH, Robbins PF, Rivoltini L, Topalian SL, Miki T, Rosenberg SA (1994a) Cloning of the gene coding for a shared human melanoma antigen recognized by autologous T cells infiltrating into tumor. Proc Natl Acad Sci USA 91:3515–3519

Kawakami Y, Eliyahu S, Sakaguchi K, Robbins PF, Rivoltini L, Yannelli JR, Appella E, Rosenberg SA (1994b) Identification of the immunodominant peptides of the MART-1 human melanoma antigen recognized by the majority of HLA-A2-restricted tumor infiltrating lymphocytes. J Exp Med 180:347–352

Knuth A, Danowski B, Oettgen HF, Old LJ (1984) T-cell-mediated cytotoxicity against autologous malignant melanoma: analysis with interleukin 2-dependent T cell cultures. Proc Natl Acad Sci USA 81:3511–3515

Knuth A, Wölfel T, Klehmann E, Boon T, Meyer zum Büschenfelde KH (1989) Cytolytic T-cell clones against an autologous human melanoma: specificity study and definition of three antigens by immunoselection. Proc Natl Acad Sci USA 86: 2804–2808

Lehmann F, Marchand M, Hainaut P, Pouillart P, Sastre X, Ikeda H, Boon T, Coulie PG (1995) Differences in the antigens recognized by cytolytic T cells on two successive metastases of a melanoma patient consistent with immunoselection. Eur J Immunol 25:340–347
Livingston PO, Shiku H, Bean MA, Oettgen HF, Old LJ (1979) Cell-mediated cytotoxicity for cultured autologous melanoma cells. Int J Cancer 24:34–44
Luscher U, Filgueira L, Juretic A, Zuber M, Luscher NJ, Heberer M, Spagnoli GC (1994) The pattern of cytokine gene expression in freshly excised human metastatic melanoma suggests a state of reversible anergy of tumor-infiltrating lymphocytes. Int J Cancer 57:612–619
Matzinger P (1994) Tolerance, danger, and the extended family. Annu Rev Immunol 12:991–1045
Mori T, Miura K, Aoki T, Mori S, Nakamura Y (1994) Frequent somatic mutation of the MTS1/CDK4I (multiple tumor suppressor/cyclin-dependent kinase 4 inhibitor) gene in esophageal squamous cell carcinoma. Cancer Res 54:3396–3397
Nanda NK, Sercarz EE (1995) Induction of anti-self-immunity to cure cancer. Cell 82: 13–17
Prehn RT (1993) Tumor immunogenicity: how far can it be pushed? Proc Natl Acad Sci USA 90:4332–4333
Ramarathinam L, Saram S, Maric M, Zhao M, Yang G, Chen L, Liu Y (1995) Multiple lineages of tumors express a common tumor antigen, P1A, but they are not cross -protected. J Immunol 155:5323–5329
Robbins PF, El-Gamil M, Li YF, Kawakami Y, Loftus D, Appella E, Rosenberg SA (1996) A mutated β-catenin gene encodes a melanoma-specific antigen recognized by tumor infiltrating lymphocytes. J Exp Med 183:1185–1192
Schirrmacher V (1992) Immunity and metastasis: in situ activation of protective T cells by virus modified cancer vaccines. Cancer Surveys 13:129–154
Seed B, Aruffo A (1987) Molecular cloning of the CD2 antigen, the T-cell erythrocyte receptor, by a rapid immunoselection procedure. Proc Natl Acad Sci USA 84:3365–3369
Skipper JCA, Hendrickson RC, Gulden PH, Brichard V, Van Pel A, Chen Y, Shabanowitz J, Wölfel T, Slingluff J, Boon T, Hunt DF, Engelhard VH (1996) An HLA-A2-restricted tyrosinase antigen on melanoma cells resulted from posttranslational modification and suggests a novel pathway for processing of membrane proteins. J Exp Med 183: 527–534
Srivastava PJ, Old LJ (1988) Individually distinct transplantation antigens of chemically induced mouse tumors. Immunol today 9:78–83
Srivastava PK, Udono H, Blachere NE, Li Z (1994) Heat shock proteins transfer peptides during antigen processing and CTL priming. Immunogenetics 39:93–98
Traversari C, Van der Bruggen P, Van den Eynde B, Hainaut P, Lemoine C, Ohta N, Old L, Boon T (1992) Transfection and expression of a gene coding for a human melanoma antigen recognized by autologous cytolytic T lymphocytes. Immunogenetics 35:145–152
Van den Eynde B, Hainaut P, Herin M, Knuth A, Lemoine C, Weynants P, Van der Bruggen P, Fauchet R, Boon T (1989) Presence on a human melanoma of multiple antigens recognized by autologous CTL. Int J Cancer 44:634–640
Visseren MJ, van Elsas A, van der Voort EI, Ressing ME, Kast WM, Schrier PI, Melief CJ (1995) CTL specific for the tyrosinase autoantigen can be induced from healthy donor blood to lyse melanoma cells. J Immunol 154:3991–3998
Wölfel T, Klehmann E, Müller C, Schütt K-H, Meyer zum Büschenfelde K-H, Knuth A (1989) Lysis of human melanoma cells by autologous cytolytic T cell clones. Identification of human histocompatibility leucocyte antigen A2 as a restriction element for three different antigens. J Exp Med 170:797–810

Wölfel T, Hauer M, Klehmann E, Brichard V, Ackermann B, Knuth A, Boon T, Meyer zum Büschenfelde K-H (1993) Analysis of antigens recognized on human melanoma cells by A2-restricted cytolytic T lymphocytes (CTL). Int J Cancer 55:237–244

Wölfel T, Schneider J, Meyer zum Büschenfelde K-H, Rammensee H-G, Rötzschke O, Falk K (1994a) Isolation of naturally processed peptides recognized by cytolytic T lymphocytes (CTL) on human melanoma cells in association with HLA-A2.1. Int J Cancer 57:413–418

Wölfel T, Van Pel A, Brichard V, Schneider J, Seliger B, Meyer zum Büschenfelde K-H, Boon T (1994b) Two tyrosinase nonapeptides recognized on HLA-A2 melanomas by autologous cytolytic T lymphocytes. Eur J Immunol. 24: 759–764

Wölfel T, Hauer M, Schneider J, Serrano M, Wölfel C, Klehmann-Hieb E, De Plaen E, Hankeln T, Meyer zum Büschenfelde K-H, Beach D (1995) A $p16^{INK4a}$-insensitive CDK4 mutant targeted by cytolytic T lymphocytes in a human melanoma. Science 269:1281–1284

Zitvogel L, Mayordomo JI, Tjandrawan T, DeLeo AB, Clarke MR, Lotze MT, Storkus WJ (1996) Therapy of murine tumors with tumor peptide-pulsed dendritic cells: dependence on T cells, B7 costimulation, and T helper cell-associated cytokines. J Exp Med 183:87–97

Zuo L, Weger J, Yang Q, Goldstein AM, Tucker MA, Walker GJ, Hayward N, Dracopoli NC (1996) Germline mutations in the $p16^{INK4a}$ binding domain of CDK4 in familial melanoma. Nat Genet 12:97–99

Deficiencies of the MHC Class I Antigen Processing and Presentation Machinery in Tumor Cells

B. Seliger and C. Huber

Introduction

The major histocompatibility complex (MHC) class I genes, which are composed of a polymorphic heavy chain noncovalently linked with β_2-microglobulin (β_2-m; Bjorkman et al. 1987), play a key role in numerous immunological processes involving the presentation of "foreign" antigens for recognition by the CD8-positive cytotoxic T lymphocytes (CTLs; Zinkernagel and Doherty 1979). This suggests that (1) cytotoxic T cells can monitor genetic changes and that (2) the MHC class I system provides an enormous diversity in potential antigenic peptide presentation including recognition of tumor cells by autologous CTL in man and animals (Boon et al. 1994).

Malignant transformation of cells which is caused by or associated with an increase in the rate of somatic mutations may provide tumor cells with mechanisms for escape from surveillance of the immune system. Indeed, human and murine tumors of various origin have been shown to express low levels of MHC class I antigens (Goodenow et al. 1985; Tanaka et al. 1985; Natali et al. 1989; Momburg et al. 1989; Cordon-Cardo et al. 1991; Garrido et al. 1993; Ferrone and Marincola 1995). Abnormalities in MHC class I antigen expression could be due to structural alterations. These include complete, allele- or locus-specific loss of the MHC class I heavy chain, and alterations in the β_2-m gene such as point mutations or partial deletions of β_2-m sequences (Garrido et al. 1993; D'Urso et al. 1991). Furthermore, dysregulation of MHC class I antigens due to transcriptional and/or posttranscriptional regulation could result in suppression of MHC class I surface expression (Table 1; Maudsley and Pound 1991; Blanchet et al 1992). Such abnormalities in class I expression are associated with resistance of tumor cells to lysis by MHC class I restricted CTLs and enhanced susceptibility to natural killer (NK)-cell-mediated lysis (Darrow et al. 1989; Wölfel et al. 1989; Ciccone et al. 1992; Salcedo et al. 1994; Bennet et al. 1995).

More recently, several groups started to analyse the MHC class I antigen presentation machinery in various human tumors as well as in *in vitro* models of viral and oncogenic transformation. Defects in such a pathway are expected to resemble lack or suppression of MHC class I antigens in their effects in regard to CTL-mediated recognition of tumor cells. Thus, characterization of functional and/or structural abnormalities in the MHC class I antigen

Symposium in Immunology VI
Eibl/Huber/Peter/Wahn (Eds.)

Table 1. Molecular mechanisms and functional consequences of MHC class I abnormalities

Lesion/mechanism	MHC class I expression	Functional implications
Nonfunctional β_2-m		
Mutations/partial deletions of promoter/gene rearrangement	Total loss	Loss of MHC class I restricted T-cell recognition Increase of NK-mediated lysis
Structural alterations		
Loss of a MHC class I haplotype	Loss of alleles	Loss of 50 % of the MHC class I repertoire
Allele loss	Decreased allele expression	Allele-specific loss
Changes in methylation pattern	Decrease or loss of MHC class I expression	Reduction of CTL-mediated lysis
Dysregulation (posttranscriptional/transcriptional)		
Increased c-myc level	Reduction in level of HLA-B and/or-C antigens	Loss/reduction of CTL mediated lysis Increased NK-sensitivity
Downregulation of alleles	Decreased allele expression	Allele-specific loss of MHC restricted recognition

presentation machinery in tumors, their role in the pathogenesis and progression of these diseases is stimulated by the current emphasis on the development and application of immunotherapeutic strategies to treat tumor patients.

The MHC Class I Antigen Presentation Machinery

The classical MHC class I antigen pathway which is operative in almost all cells monitors endogenously synthesized proteins (Townsend and Bodmer 1989; Goldberg and Rock 1992; Rivett 1993; Barber and Parham 1994). Proteins are rapidly degraded by a soluble ATP-dependent process that involves ubiquitin and the 26S proteolytic complex. Proteins are marked for rapid degradation by conjugation with multiple ubiquitin molecules, leading to hydrolysis by the 26S proteasome which contains multiple peptidase activities (Hershko and Cienchover 1992; Goldberg 1995). Some of the yielded peptides are transported into the endoplasmic reticulum (ER) by an ATP-/NTP-dependent heterodimeric complex, where they bind to the newly assembled MHC class I molecules and are transported via the trans-Golgi to the cell surface (Schumacher et al. 1991; Hill and Ploegh 1995). Some peptides may also be generated or modified by proteolysis in the ER prior to presentation (Roelse et al. 1994). The immune system uses this pathway to screen the cytosol for abnormal proteins. Peptides derived from autologous proteins are usually ignored due to self tolerance, whereas foreign peptides, e.g., viral or mutated gene products, may be recognized by CTL.

The characterization of cells with defects in the antigen presentation machinery has led to the identification of four components, which have been named the low molecular mass proteins, LMP-2 and LMP-7, and the transporters associated with antigen processing, TAP-1 and TAP-2.

The LMP-2 and LMP-7 genes are located in the MHC class II locus and their gene products were identified as two subunits of the multicatalytic proteasome complex (Brown et al.1991; Glynne et al. 1991; Ortiz-Navarette et al. 1991). Although still controversially discussed, several lines of evidence suggest a role for LMP-2 and LMP-7 in the antigen processing (Arnold et al. 1992; Momburg et al. 1992, Michalek et al. 1993). These include the effects of different protease inhibitors on the generation of MHC class I-presented peptides (Rock et al. 1994), the involvement of the proteasome mediated ubiquitin-dependent proteolysis in antigen presentation (Townsend et al. 1989) as well as the reduced MHC class I surface expression in LMP-2/ LMP-7 knock-out mice (Fehling et al. 1994; van Kaer et al. 1992). Interferon-γ (IFN-γ) treatment modulates the proteolytic activity of the proteasomes and induces the transcription of both LMP genes (Yang et al. 1992; Driscoll et al. 1993; Epperson et al. 1993; Gaczynska et al, 1993; Seliger et al. 1996). Furthermore, peptide presentation could be restored in LMP defect mutants by LMP gene transfer (Cerundolo et al. 1995; Rotem-Yeduhar et al. 1996). Like the LMP genes, TAP-1 and TAP-2 reside in the MHC class II locus and are polymorphic (Deverson et al. 1990; Spies et al. 1990; Trowsdale et al. 1990). Amino acid sequence comparison revealed that TAP proteins exhibit a high degree of homology to the large family of ABC transporters (Higgins 1994), possessing two stretches of six to eight membrane spanning regions and a C-terminal highly conserved nucleotide binding domain (Monaco et al. 1990; Spies et al. 1990; Uebel et al. 1995). TAP-1 and TAP-2 form a heterodimer located in the membrane of the ER and cis-Golgi. In the ER, TAP-1 is directly associated with the MHC class I heterodimer (Suh et al. 1994). There are different lines of evidence for the involvement of the TAP-1/TAP-2 dimer in the translocation of antigenic peptides from the cytosol into the lumen of the ER (Hill and Ploegh 1995): (1) restoration of correct antigen presentation in mutants transfected with TAP genes (Spies and DeMars 1991; Attaya et al. 1992); (2) peptide translocation assays using permeabilized cells (Androlewicz et al. 1993; Neefjes et al. 1993) or microsomes prepared from mammalian cells (Shepherd et al.1993); and (3) inhibition of peptide transport by mutations in the TAP molecule (Kovacsovics-Banikowski and Rock 1995). The affinity and efficiency of the TAP-mediated peptide transport is dependent on the length and sequence of the peptides as well as the TAP-polymorphism (Momburg et al. 1994; Schumacher et al. 1994; van Endert et al. 1994; Uebel et al. 1995).

A prerequisite for optimal MHC class I antigen presentation is an effective peptide transport via the TAP heterodimer. Thus, a lack of or reduced TAP function results in defective assembly and loading of MHC class I molecules with peptides. As a consequence MHC class I surface expression is low, since only the trimeric complex consisting of MHC heavy and light chain molecules associated with the peptide is stably expressed on the cell membrane (Ljunggren et al. 1990; Goldberg and Rock 1992; Yewdell and Bennink 1992).

Indeed, suppression of MHC class I surface expression was observed in tumor cells with deletions in the MHC class II locus or mutations in the TAP gene and in TAP-/- mice (Ljunggren and Kärre 1985; van Kaer et al. 1992). In these cells, MHC class I surface expression could be enhanced by the addition of exogenous MHC class I binding peptides, by incubation at low, unphysiological temperature and by TAP gene transfer (Ljunggren et al. 1990; Townsend et al. 1989; Spies and DeMars 1991).

Effects of Viral Transformation on the MHC Class I Antigen Processing Machinery

Adenovirus (Ad) transformed cells have been widely employed as model systems for the analysis of the direct correlation between tumorigenicity and lack of host immune responses due to decreased MHC class I surface expression (Schrier et al. 1983; Eager et al. 1985). Ad12-mediated downregulation of MHC class I expression seemed to occur at both the transcriptional and posttranscriptional level (Ackrill and Blair 1988; Shemesh et al. 1991; Friedman and Ricciardi 1988; Shemesh and Ehrlich 1993). Rotem-Yeduhar and coworkers (1994, 1996) demonstrated that Ad12 affects MHC class I antigen levels by downregulating the expression of the peptide transporters and proteasome subunits. This results in a reduced availability of relevant peptides for stable assembly and transport of class I molecules to the cell surface. Re-expression of TAP and LMP in Ad12-transformed cells resulted in a complete reconstitution of MHC class I surface expression. However, efficient transport of MHC class I molecules could only be obtained by IFN-γ treatment.

Downregulation of MHC class I surface expression has also been observed in a number of cervical carcinomas containing the human papilloma virus 16/18 (Cromme et al. 1993) and was associated with a loss of TAP-1 expression (Cromme et al. 1994). Furthermore, Burkitt lymphomas containing Epstein-Barr virus (EBV) sequences are deficient in MHC class I expression due to the inability to process intracellular antigenic determinants (Khanna et al. 1994; Rowe et al. 1995). In Herpes simplex virus-infected cells, the cytoplasmic protein ICP47 efficiently inhibits the peptide transport due to its complex formation with TAP (Früh et al. 1995). The direct suppression of peptide translocation by the ICP47 protein seems to be one mechanism for virus-infected cells to escape immune surveillance. These data raise the possibility that DNA viruses affect not only the expression of MHC class I molecules, but also other components of the antigen processing machinery. One can speculate that a similar mechanism – the induction of specific TAP inhibitors during neoplastic transformation – may be a specific event in the development of tumor cells.

Characterisation of TAP and LMP Expression in Renal Cell Carcinoma Cell Lines

In order to study the MHC class I antigen processing machinery, 11 human renal cell carcinoma (RCC) cell lines established from primary tumors were analyzed for steady state mRNA levels and protein expression of MHC class I, TAP, and LMP genes. Northern blot analysis revealed specific transcripts for HLA class I heavy and light chain and TAP-1, TAP-2, LMP-2, and LMP-7 mRNA in all RCC lines. mRNA expression of these genes was quite heterogenous among the RCC lines, but in most individual cell lines, the proteasome subunits, transporters, and the MHC class I molecules were coordinately expressed (Fig. 1; Seliger et al. 1996).

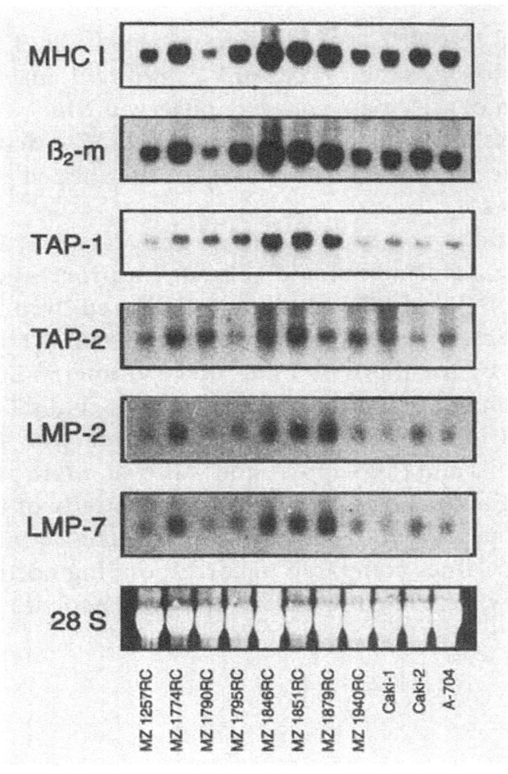

Fig. 1 Northern blot analysis of different RCC lines. Total cellular RNA from RCC lines was subjected to Northern blot analysis. The blots were sequentially rehybridized to cDNA probes of MHC class I heavy chain, β_2-m TAP-1, TAP-2, LMP-2, and LMP-7

Table 2. Reduced TAP, LMP and MHC class I expression in renal cell carcinoma and their modulation

Cell lines	Expression			Modulation	
	TAP	LMP	MHC I	IFN-sensitivity	MHC class I stabilization
MZ1257RC	+	+	+	+ + +	+ +
MZ1774RC	+ +	+ +	+ +	+ +	+
MZ1790RC	+	(+)	+	+ + +	+ +
MZ1795RC	+	+	+	+ +	+ +
MZ1846RC	+ +	+ +	+ +	+ +	+
MZ1851RC	+ +	+ +	+ +	+ +	+
MZ1851LN	(+)	(+)	+	+ +	+ + +
MZ1879RC	+ +	+ +	+ +	+ +	+
MZ1940RC	(+)	+	+	+ +	+ +
MZ1851NN	+ + +	n.d.	+ + +	+	–
MZ1879NN	+ +	n.d.	+ + +	+	–
MZ1940NN	+ +	n.d.	+ + +	+	–

+ + +, high level of expression/modulation; + +, intermediate level of expression/modulation; +, low level of expression/modulation; (+) very little if any expression/modulation; –, no expression/modulation; n.d., no data.

In parallel, the TAP, LMP, and the MHC class I protein expression of the RCC lines were determined by flow cytometry and/or Western blot analysis (Table 2). Again, distinct protein density patterns were observed which correlated with their transcript levels. These data suggest a parallel regulation of steady state mRNA and protein levels of the genes coding for the antigen presentation machinery in RCC lines.

To investigate whether the modulation of MHC class I antigens, TAP, and LMP molecules occurs during transformation and subsequent progression, normal epithelial kidney cells (NN) and RCC cell lines established from the primary tumor (RC) and in one case from a lymph node metastasis (LN) of the same patient were analyzed by Northern blot and flow cytometry. Both the mRNA and protein expression of MHC class I heavy and light chain, TAP, and LMP was strongly reduced in primary RCC lines compared with the corresponding normal kidney cells and this suppression was even more pronounced in the metastatic cell line (Table 2). In addition, the activity of the TAP molecules as measured by peptide translocation assays was also markedly diminished in primary RCC lines compared to corresponding normal kidney cells and was further downregulated in cells of the metastatic lesion (Fig. 2).

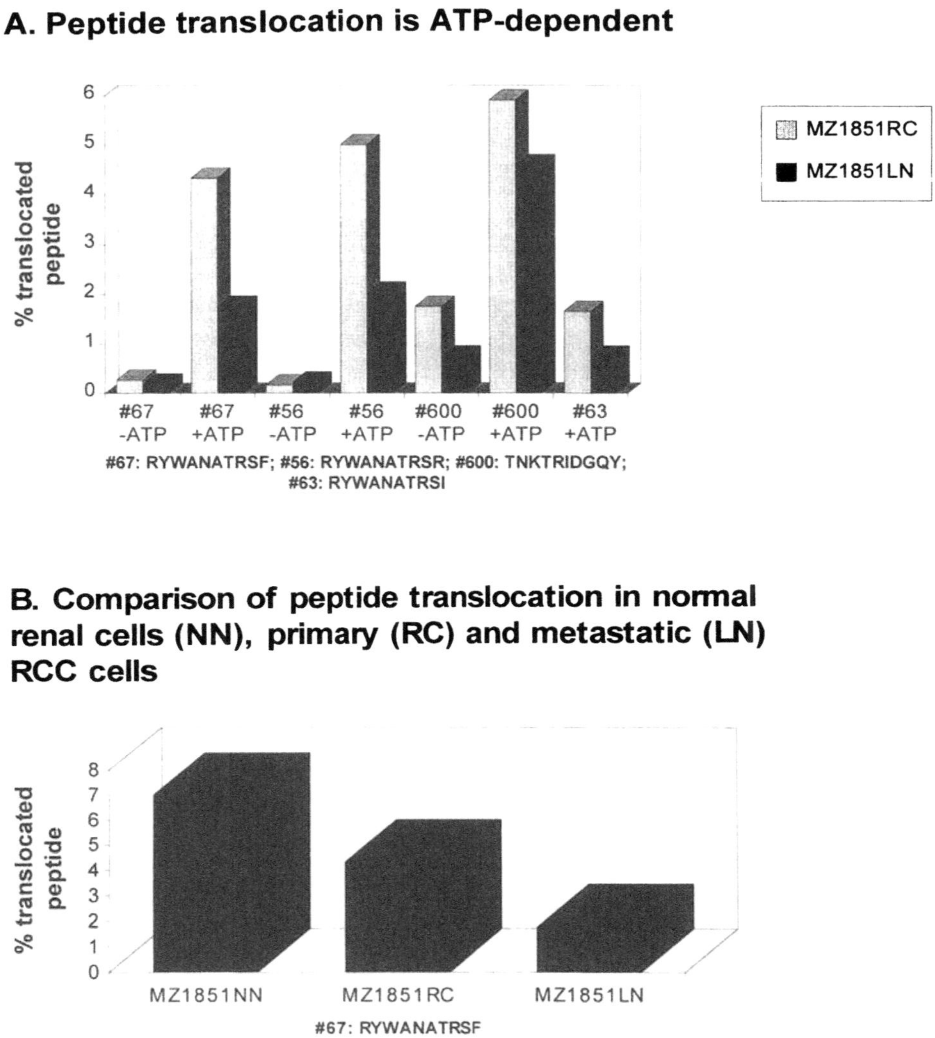

Fig. 2 **A.** TAP-dependent peptide translocation of input peptides. The peptide #67 (RYWANATRSF) was translocated in the presence and absence of ATP by streptolysin-O-permeabilized MZ1851RC and MZ1851LN cells. Translocated peptides were isolated with ConA Sepharose, quantitated and expressed as percentage of input peptide. Similar results were obtained with the 10-mer peptides #63 (RYWABATRSI) and #600 (TNKTRIDGQY) #67, RYWANATRSF; #56, RYWANATRSR. **B.** Comparison of peptide translocation in normal renal cells (**NN**), primary (**RC**), and metastatic (**LN**) cells. #67, RYWANATRSF

Modulation of MHC Class I Surface Expression in RCC Lines Using Different Culture Conditions

The expression of the heavy chain/β_2-m dimers on the surface of the TAP defect mutants was unstable at physiological temperature due to dissociation into their component proteins which could no longer be detected by conformation-specific antibodies. To determine the stability or instability of the three-dimensional MHC class I structure at the cell surface, RCC lines were cultivated in parallel for 24 h at low (26 °C) and physiological (37 °C) temperature. MHC class I surface expression was assessed by flow cytometry, and stability indices were calculated by dividing values of specific fluorescence intensity obtained at 26 °C with those of cells kept at 37 °C (Table 2). Cells without TAP/LMP deficiencies, e.g., normal renal cells, fibroblasts, and EBV-transformed B-cells as well as defect mutants, served as controls. The results revealed the existence of two different phenotypes of RCC cell lines: group I displayed temperature-stable MHC class I surface expression associated with high and in most cases coordinated expression of MHC class I heavy and light chain, TAP, and LMP transcripts and proteins. Group II demonstrated a marked MHC class I instability at 37 °C associated with low but coordinated expression of the respective transcripts and proteins.

It has recently been shown that MHC class I surface expression of cells lacking or expressing reduced amounts of TAP and/or LMP proteins could be increased by the addition of exogenous MHC clas I-binding peptides. For example, a HLA-A2-binding peptide was able to reconstitute HLA-A2 surface expression on the TAP-deficient T2 cells (Townsend et al. 1989; Wölfel et al. 1994). To determine whether this was also the case in RCC cell lines, especially those of group II, the HLA-A2-expressing RCC cells were cultured in the presence of the HLA-A2-binding peptide. An H-2L^d-binding CMV peptide served as a negative control. MHC class I membrane expression of group II, but not of group I RCC cells could be stabilized by incubation with specific MHC class I-binding peptides. Furthermore, MHC class I surface expression of normal renal cells was not affected under these culture conditions. These results demonstrated that the peptide transporters and proteasome subunits are important for a stable and efficient MHC class I surface expression of RCC cells. However, it has still to be determined whether such defects in the antigen processing machinery represent one of the mechanisms whereby RCC escapes immune surveillance.

Interferons are known inducers of the transcription of both MHC class I heavy chain and β_2-m (Ting and Baldwin 1993) leading to increased class I mRNA and protein levels. The effect of IFNs on the expression of MHC, TAP, and LMP was analyzed in representative RCC lines. IFN-α and particularly IFN-γ stimulation increased MHC class I, TAP, and LMP transcript and protein levels of RCC lines, but with a distinct IFN response kinetic (Fig 3). Similar results were obtained by Epperson and colleagues (1993) who demonstrated an IFN-γ-mediated upregulation of TAP and LMP transcript and protein levels prior to MHC class I induction in endothelial cell lines. Both cytokines had no additional effect on the stability of MHC class I surface expression in RCC lines. The recent characterization of the dual TAP-1/LMP-2 promoter demonstrated a coordinate regulation of these genes, which further suggested a functional linkage between both gene products (Wright et al. 1995).

The analysis of the MHC class I antigen presentation machinery in human RCC lines and their normal counterparts as well as its modulation by different experimental approaches suggest (1) that malignant transformation and subsequent *in vivo* selection of renal tubular cells can lead to the recovery of carcinoma cells which stably express an immune escape phenotype; (2) that deficiencies associated with this phenotype involve all levels of the MHC class I restricted antigen presentation machinery; (3) that defects in TAP and/or LMP expression are more pronounced in metastatic cells; and (4) that abnormalities in the MHC class I antigen processing pathway are at least partially restored by IFN treatment.

Defects in the Antigen Processing Machinery: A General Mechanism in Human Tumors?

In a number of human tumors of distinct origin, a lack of or reduced MHC class I surface expression was observed and seemed to be one strategy of tumor cells to evade CTL-mediated recognition and elimination (Ruiz-Cabello et al. 1991; Garrido et al. 1993; Ferrone and Marincola 1995). Suppression of MHC class I surface expression could be caused by abnormalities in the expression of MHC class I antigens due to structural alterations and dysregulation of heavy and light chain molecules (Table 1). More recently, analyses of TAP and LMP were performed using a variety of human tumor cell lines and tumor lesions (Table 3). The results of these analyses suggest that the defects in the components of the antigen processing machinery found in RCC resemble those described in other tumor types.

Whether poor MHC class I surface expression is accompanied by a significantly decreased capacity to present endogenously synthesized proteins was first analyzed in small cell lung carcinoma (SCLC) cell lines (Restifo et al. 1993). Different SCLC lines were infected with a recombinant vaccinia virus (Vac) to transiently express the H-2 K^d molecules and then tested for lysis by Vac-specific CTL. The experiments showed that some SCLC cells failed to process endogenously synthesized proteins for presentation to H-2 K^d-restricted, Vac-specific T cells, suggesting that peptides were not available for binding to nascent MHC class I molecules in the ER. The poor antigen processing of SCLC cells seemed to be due to downregulation of TAP and LMP steady state mRNA levels (Restifo et al. 1993).

Table 3. Downregulation of TAP, LMP, and MHC class I antigens in human tumors

A: Analysis of tumor sections

		% of cases with downregulated expression			
		Primary		Metastasis	
Tumor type	No. of cases	MHC I	TAP	MHC I	TAP
Melanoma	32	n.d.	16	n.d.	22
Breast	63	33	33	44	44
Colorectal cancer	81	n.d.	14	n.d.	n.d.
Cervical cancer	76	49	49	n.d.	n.d.

B. Analysis of human tumor cell lines

		Suppression of antigen processing genes			
Tumor type	No. of cases	MHC I	TAP-1	TAP-2	LMP-2/-7
Melanoma	9	?	5/ 9	5/ 9	7/ 9
Small cell lung	3	n.d.	3/ 3	3/ 3	3/ 3
Prostate cancer	5	1/ 5	n.d.	2/ 5	n.d.
Burkitt lymphoma	8	n.d.	8/ 8	7/ 8	0/ 8
Renal cell cancer	12	12/12	12/12	12/12	12/12

n.d., no data.

Comparable results were obtained in Burkitt lymphoma (BL) cell lines. Some BL lines expressed low levels of MHC class I antigens on the cell surface which also reflected a suppression of TAP transcript and protein production (Rowe et al. 1995). Restoration of the immunogenicity of BL cells were obtained by insertion of an ER signal sequence facilitating the transport of peptide epitopes (Khanna et al. 1994). Furthermore, treatment of BL and SCLC cells with IFN-γ restored the antigen processing function as measured by the ability of these cells to present endogenously expressed viral antigens to the CTLs (Restifo et al. 1993; Rowe et al. 1995).

Human metastatic prostate cancer cells can escape T-cell recognition via distinct mechanisms of defective MHC class I assembly (Sanda et al. 1995). Some prostate cancer cells underexpressed TAP-2 mRNA despite abundant MHC class I antigen expression. The resistance of these cells to CTL-mediated lysis could be restored by IFN-γ treatment. In contrast, the prostate cancer cell line LNCaP had competent antigen transport, but deficient MHC class I assembly which was specifically related to the abnormal functioning of the MHC class I heavy chain molecules. Thus, Sanda et al. (1995) demonstrated a novel regulatory defect among cancers showing suppression of TAP-2 expression independent of MHC class I heavy chain expression.

In melanoma cell lines as well as in surgically removed melanoma lesions, a loss of MHC class I antigen expression occurs frequently in primary lesions and even more often in metastasis (D'Urso et al. 1991; Garrido et al. 1993; Ferrone and Marincola 1995). In comparison to EBV-transformed B lymphocytes from melanoma patients, melanoma cell lines expressed low levels of LMP and TAP transcripts and proteins (Hicklin et al. 1996; Maeurer et al. 1996; Seliger et al. 1996). Furthermore, most of the melanoma cell lines displayed a significant instability of MHC class I antigen expression at 37 °C, which could be corrected by incubation of cells at low temperature. These data suggest that downregulation of the MHC class I surface expression is caused by a lack of peptides in the ER. Ferrone and coworkers also analyzed LMP and TAP protein expression in surgically removed melanoma lesions. Immunohistochemical stainings revealed a downregulation of LMP-2 and LMP-7 expression in about 20 % and 6 % of primary melanoma lesions respectively, and in about 40 % and 12 % of metastatic lesions. With regard to peptide transporters, approximately 15 % of primary melanomas and 22 % of metastases failed to express TAP. Thus, the frequency of deficiencies in TAP and LMP expression seemed to be associated with the development and progression of this malignancy. Similar results were obtained by immunohistochemical staining of primary breast carcinomas and related lymph node metastasis as well as colorectal cancer (Kaklamanis et al. 1994, 1995). Although less frequent, a loss of MHC class I expression in breast and colon cancer patients was accompanied by a defective TAP-1 expression in up to 20 % of patients. Thus, the incidence of deficiencies in TAP and LMP expression seemed to be associated with development and progression of malignancies. Restoration of TAP and LMP function has been accomplished by IFN-γ treatment and is sufficient to regain CTL-mediated recognition of tumor cells in most cases studied. These data also provide evidence that patients exhibiting low or no MHC class I expression on tumors due to TAP/LMP defects may clinically benefit from cytokine treatment if tumor regression can be mediated by immune effector cells.

Alternative Immune Recognition of TAP Deficient Cells

Presentation of cytosolic peptides to MHC class I-restricted T cells can also be detected in the absence of TAP (Hosken and Bevan 1992; Zweerink et al. 1993) and can be improved by attachment of a signal sequence for ER translocation. It has been shown that cell surface expression of HLA-A2 is much less dependent on TAP than other alleles. Analysis of peptides eluted from HLA-A2 molecules in TAP-defective cells revealed that most peptides were derived from signal sequences (Wei and Cresswell 1992, Henderson et al. 1992). Thus, peptide leader sequences cleaved in the ER have the capacity to provide an epitope for HLA-A2-restricted T-cell recognition (Gueguen et al.

1994). In the case of tyrosinase, two nonapeptides are recognized by autologous CTLs, one of which is derived from the putative signal sequence of tyrosinase (Wölfel et al. 1994).

Cells could also use different strategies to circumvent the need for MHC class I-mediated immune recognition. An alternative tumor-directed cellular response involves NK-cells. In general tumor cells with reduced or lack of MHC class I surface expression are good targets for NK-cells whereas the presence of specific MHC alleles prevents NK-cell recognition. Thus, TAP deficient cells are highly susceptible to NK-cell-mediated lysis (Salcedo et al. 1994). Reversal of the NK-sensitive phenotype was achieved by TAP gene transfer. Besides NK-cell recognition, other structures, e.g., MHC class II molecules, CD1, and heat shock proteins (HSPs), which are also TAP-independent could be presented to immune cells. For instance in melanoma, MHC class II-restricted tumor-reactive CTL recognition has been detected. In the case of human CD1 molecules presenting non-peptide antigens it has to be investigated whether these structures are able to induce cell-mediated immunity. Furthermore, it has been suggested that HSPs may present target structures in antitumor responses.

Summary and Conclusions

Although it was recently found that exogenous antigens can be presented by MHC class I molecules, the endogenously synthesized peptides constitute the major source of peptides for MHC class I-restricted presentation to CTL (Rock 1996). Proper assembly of MHC class I molecules and their transport to the cell surface requires the binding of peptides. Cytosolic peptides are delivered into the ER via the NTP-dependent TAP complex. Cells with genetic alterations and/or dysregulation, especially of the TAP genes, usually lack or express low levels of MHC class I antigens on the cell surface and therefore fail to generate an effective T-cell response.

The analysis of the antigen processing machinery demonstrated a loss or downregulation of the peptide transporter genes TAP-1 and TAP-2 and the proteasome subunits LMP-2 and LMP-7 in a variety of tumor cell lines and tumor specimens of distinct origin. This was found to result in low or no MHC class I antigen expression. These data suggest that TAP and LMP deficiencies seem to play a critical role in the development and progression of different neoplastic diseases due to the aberrant functioning of T-cell-mediated immunity.

If such functional defects of the antigen processing/presentation machinery represent a general mechanism of tumor cells to evade immune surveillance, this should be considered in the development of future immunotherapies. The findings described here provide a rational basis for the development of innovative immunotherapies. The successful implementation of

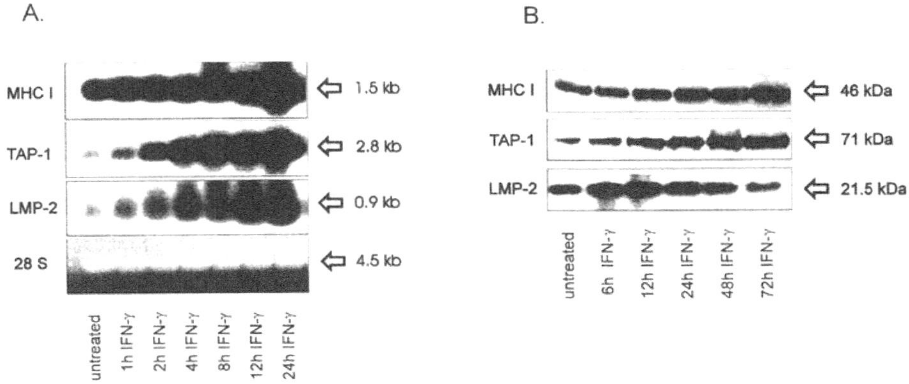

Fig. 3 IFN-γ mediated induction of MHC class I antigens, TAP-1, and LMP-2 in renal cell carcinoma cell lines. **A.** 20 μg total cellular RNA from MZ1257RC cells, either untreated or treated with IFN-γ (20 ng/ml) for the time points indicated was subjected to Northern blot analysis. The blots were sequentially hybridized to cDNA probes for MHC class I, TAP-1, and LMP-2. **B.** Western blot analysis of MZ1257RC cells. 20 μg protein from untreated as well as IFN-γ treated cells was subjected to Western blot analysis. The blots were treated with the primary antibodies TAP-1 (mAb 148.3), LMP-2 and HLA-A, -B, -C (W6/32) over night and then with alkaline phosphatase conjugated (for TAP 1, MHC I) or peroxidase conjugated secondary antibodies (for LMP-2) for 15 to 60 min and analysed according to the Amersham enhanced chemiluminescence system (ECL; Amersham, UK)

T-cell-based immunotherapy in cancer patients warrants careful examination of the patients' tumor in order to define the most effective therapy. Future research in this field should include a monitoring of the MHC class I antigen pathway and its modulation by cytokine treatment, screening for costimulatory and adhesion molecules which are essential for an effective T-cell response as well as a search for new approaches to circumvent the sole reliance on MHC class I-mediated tumor-cell recognition, e.g. the identification of novel target structures recognized by alternative immune effector cells.

References

Ackrill AM, Blair GE (1988) Regulation of the major histocompatibility class I gene expression at the level of transcription in highly oncogenic adenovirus transformed rat cells. Oncogene 3:483–487

Androlewicz MJ, Ortmann B, Van Endert PM, Spies T, Cresswell P (1993) Characteristics of peptide and major histocompatibility complex class-I β_2-microglobulin binding to the transporters associated with antigen-processing (tap1 and tap2). Proc Natl Acad Sci USA 91:12716–12720

Arnold DJ, Driscoll M, Androlewicz M, Hughes E, Cresswell P, Spies T (1992) Proteasome subunits encoded in the MHC are not generally required for the processing of peptides bound by MHC class I molecules. Nature 360:171–174

Attaya M, Jameson S, Martinez E, Hermel E, Aldrich C, Forman J, Fischer-Lindahl K, Bevan MJ, Monaco JJ (1992) Ham-2 corrects the class I antigen-processing defect in RMA-S cells. Nature 355:647–649

Barber L, Parham P (1994) The essence of epitopes. J Exp Med 180:1191–1194

Bennet M, Lawrence YY, Stoneman E, Rembecki RM, Mathew PA, Fisher-Lindahl K, Kumar V (1995) Hybrid resistance: "negative" and "positive" signaling of murine natural killer cells. Semin Immunol 7:121–127

Bjorkman PJ, Saper MA, Saraoui B, Bennett WS, Strominger JL, Wiley DC (1987) Structure of the human MHC class I histocompatibility antigens. Nature 329:512–518

Blanchet O, Bourge J-F, Zinszner H, Israel A, Kourilsky P, Dausset J, Degos L, Paul P (1992) Altered binding of regulatory factors to HLA class I enhancer sequence in human tumor cells lacking class I antigen expression. Proc Natl Acad Sci USA 89:3488–3492

Boon T, Cerrottini JC, van den Eynde B, van der Bruggen P, van der Pel A (1994) Tumor antigens recognized by T-lymphocytes. Annu Rev Immunol 12:337–365

Brown MC, Driscoll J, Monaco JJ (1991) Structural and serological similarity of MHC-linked LMP and proteasome (multicatalytic proteinase) complexes. Nature 353:355–357

Cerundolo V, Kelly A, Elliott T, Trowsdale J, Townsend A (1995) Genes encoded in the major histocompatibility complex affecting the generation of peptides for TAP transport. Eur J Immunol 25:554–562

Ciccone E, Pende D, Viale O, Di Donato C, Orengo AM, Biassoni R, Verdiani S, Amoroso A, Moretta A, Moretta L (1992) Involvement of HLA class I alleles in NK cell-specific function: expression of HLA-Cw3 confers selective protection from lysis by alloreactive clones displaying a defined specifity (specifity 2). J Exp Med 176:963–971

Cordon-Cardo C, Fuks Z, Drobnjak M, Moreno C, Eisenbach L, Feldman M (1991) Expression of HLA-A, B, C antigens on primary and metastatic tumor cell populations of human carcinomas. Cancer Res 51:6372–6380

Cromme FV, Meijer CJLM, Snidjers PJF, Uyterlinde U, Kenemans P, Helmerhorst T, Stern PL, van der Brule AJC, Walboomers JJ (1993) Analysis of MHC class I and class II expression in relation to presence of HPV genotypes in premalignant and malignant cervical lesions. Br J Cancer 67:1372–1380

Cromme FV, Airey J, Heemels MT, Ploegh H, Keating PJ, Stern PL, Meijer CJLM, Walboomers JMM (1994) Loss of transporter protein, encoded by the TAP-1 gene, is highly correlated with loss of HLA expression in cervical carcinomas. J Exp Med 179:335–340

Darrow TL, Slingluff CL, Siegler HF (1989) The role of HLA class I antigens in recognition of melanoma cells by tumor specific cytolytic T Iymphocytes. J Immunol 142:3329–3335

Deverson EV, Gow IR, Coadwell WJ, Monaco JJ, Butcher GW, Howard JC (1990) MHC class II region encoding proteins are related to the multidrug resistance family of transmembrane transporters. Nature 348:738–741

Driscoll J, Brown MG, Finley D, Monaco JJ (1993) MHC-linked LMP gene products specifically alter peptidase activities of the proteasome. Nature 365:262–264

D'Urso CM, Wang ZG, Cao Y, Tatake R, Zeff RA, Ferrone S (1991) Lack of HLA class I antigen expression by cultured melanoma FO-1 cells due to a defect in β_2-m gene expression. J Clin Invest 87:284–292

Eager K, Williams J, Breiding D, Pans S, Knowles B, Appella E, Ricciardi RP (1985) Expression of histocompatibility antigens H-2K, -D, and -L is reduced in adenovirus 12 transformed mouse cells and is restored by IFN. Proc Natl Acad Sci USA 82:5525–5529

Epperson DE, Arnold D, Spies T, Cresswell P, Pober JS, Johnson DR (1992) Cytokines increase transporter in antigen processing-1 expression more rapidly than HLA class I expression in endothelial cells. J Immunol 149:3297–3301
Fehling HJ, Swat W, Laplace C, Kühn R, Rajewsky K, Müller U, von Böhmer H (1994) MHC class I expression in mice lacking the proteasome subunit LMP-7. Science 265:1234–1237
Ferrone S, Marincola FM (1995) Loss of HLA class I antigens by melanoma cells: molecular mechanisms, functional significance and clinical relevance. Immunol Today 16:487–494
Friedman DJ, Ricciardi RP (1988) Adenovirus type 12 E1A gene represses accumulation of MHC class I mRNAs at the level of transcription. Virol 165:303–305
Früh K, Ahn K, Djaballah H, Sempé P, van Endert PM, Tampé R, Peterson PA, Yang Y (1995) A viral inhibitor of peptide transporters for antigen presentation. Nature 375:415–418
Gaczynska M, Rock KL, Goldberg AL (1993) Interferon-gamma and expression of MHC genes regulate peptide hydrolysis by proteasomes. Nature 365:264–267
Garrido F, Cabrera T, Concha A, Glew S, Ruiz-Cabello F, Stern PL (1993) Natural history of HLA expression during tumour development. Immunol Today 14:491–499
Glynne R, Powis SH, Beck S, Kelly A, Kerr LA, Trowsdale J (1991) A proteasome-related gene between the two ABC transporter loci in the class II region of the human MHC. Nature 353:357–360
Goldberg AL (1995) Functions of the proteasome: the lysis at the end of the tunnel. Science 268:522–523
Goldberg AL, Rock KL (1992) Proteolysis, proteasomes and antigen presentation. Nature 357:375–379
Goodenow RS, Vogel JM, Linsk RL (1985) Histocompatibility antigens on murine tumors. Science 230:777–783
Gueguen M, Biddison WE, Long EO (1994) T-cell recognition of an HLA-A2 restricted epitope derived from a cleaved signal sequence. J Exp Med 180:1989–1994
Hämmerling GJ, Klar D, Pulm W, Momburg F, Moldenhauer G (1987) The influence of MHC class I antigens on tumor growth and metastasis. Biochim Biophys Acta 179:245–259
Heemels MT, Ploegh HL (1994) Substrate-specificity of allelic variants of the tap peptide transporter. Immunity 1:775–784
Henderson RA, Michel H, Sakaguchi K, Shabanowitz J, Appella E, Hunt DF, Engelhard VH (1992) HLA-A2.1 associated peptides from a mutant cell line: a second pathway of antigen presentation. Science 255:1264–1266
Hershko A, Cienchover A (1992) The ubiquitin system for protein degradation. Annu Rev Biochem 61:761–807
Hicklin DJ, Kageshita T, Dellaratta DV, Boccaletti V, Ferrone S (1996) Defects in HLA class I antigen presentation machinery in melanoma cells. (In press)
Higgins CF (1994) Introduction: the ABC transporter channel superfamily: an overview. Semin Cell Biol 4:1–5
Hill A, Ploegh H (1995) Getting the inside out: The transporter associated with antigen processing and the presentation of viral antigen. Proc Natl Acad Sci USA 92:341–342
Hosken NA, Bevan MJ (1992) An endogenous antigenic peptide bypasses the class I antigen presentation defect in RMA-S. J Exp Med 175:719–729
Kaklamanis L, Townsend A, Doussis-Anagnostopouloou IA, Mortensen N, Harris AL, Gatter KC (1994) Loss of major histocompatibility complex-encoded transporter associated with antigen presentation (TAP) in colorectal cancer. Am J Pathol 145:505–509

Kaklamanis L, Leek R, Koukourakis M, Gatter KC, Harris AL (1995). Loss of transporter in antigen processing 1 transport protein and major histocompatibility complex class I molecules in primary and metastatic breast cancer. Cancer Res 55:5191–5194

Khanna R, Burrows SR, Argaet V, Moss D (1994) Endoplasmic reticulum signal sequence facilitated transport of peptide epitopes restores immunogenicity of an antigen processing defective tumor cell line. Int Immunol 6:639–645

Kovacsovics-Banikowski M, Rock KL (1995) A phagosome to cytosol pathway for exogenous antigens presented on MHC class I molecules. Science 267:243–246

Ljunggren HG, Kärre K (1985) Host resistance directed selectively against H-2 deficient lymphoma variants: analysis of the mechanism. J Exp Med 1162:1745–1749

Ljunggren HG, Stam NJ, Öhlen C, Neefjes JJ, Hoglund P, Heemels MT, Bastin J, Schumacher TNM, Townsend A, Kärre K, Ploegh HL (1990) Empty MHC class I molecules come out in the cold. Nature 346:476–480

Maudsley DJ, Pound JD (1991) Modulation of MHC antigen expression by viruses and oncogenes. Immunol Today 12:429–431

Michalek MT, Grant EP, Gramm C, Goldberg AL, Rock KL (1993) A role for the ubiquitin-dependent proteolytic pathway in MHC class I restricted antigen presentation. Nature 363:552–554

Momburg F, Ziegler A, Harpprecht J, Möller P, Moldenhauer G, Hämmerling GJ (1989) Selective loss of HLA-A or HLA-B antigen expression in colon carcinoma. J Immunol 142:352–358

Momburg F, Ortiz-Navarette V, Neefjes J, Goulmy E, van de Wal Y, Spits H, Powis SJ, Butcher GW, Howard JC, Walden P, Hämmerling GJ (1992) Proteasome subunits encoded by the major histocompatibility complex are not essential for antigen presentation. Nature 360:174–177

Momburg F, Roelse J, Hämmerling GJ, Neefjes JJ (1994) Peptide size selection by the major histocompatibility complex encoded peptide transporter. J Exp Med 179:1613–1623

Monaco JJ, Cho S, Attaya M (1990) Transport protein genes in the murine MHC: possible implications for antigen processing. Science 250:1723–1726

Müller KM, Ebensberger C, Tampé R (1994) Nucleotide binding to the hydrophilic C-terminal domain of the transporter associated with antigen processing TAP. J Biol Chem 269:14032–14037

Natali PG, Nicotra MR, Bigotti A, Venturo I, Marcenaro L, Giacomini P, Russo C (1989) Selective changes in the expression of HLA class I polymorphic determinants in human solid tumors. Proc Natl Acad Sci USA 86:6719–6723

Neefjes JJ, Momburg F, Hämmerling G (1993) Selective and ATP-dependent translocation of peptides by the MHC-encoded transporter. Science 261:769–771

Ortiz-Navarette V, Seelig A, Gernold M, Frentzel S, Kloetzel JM, Hämmerling GJ (1991) Subunit of the "20S" proteasome (multicatalytic proteinase) encoded by the major histocompatibility complex. Nature 353:662–664

Restifo NP, Esquivel F, Kawakami Y, Yewdell JW, Mule JJ, Rosenberg SA, Bennink JR (1993) Identification of human cancers deficient in antigen processing. J Exp Med 177:265–272

Rivett AJ (1993) Proteasomes: multicatalytic proteinase complexes. Biochem J 291:1–10

Rock KL (1996) A new foreign policy: MHC class I molecules monitor the outside world. Immunol Today 17:131–137

Rock KL, Gramm C, Rothstein L, Clark K, Stein R, Dick L, Hwang D, Goldberg AL (1994) Inhibitors of the proteasome block the degradation of most cell proteins and the generation of peptides presented on MHC class I molecules. Cell 78:761–771

Roelse J, Grommé M, Momburg F, Hämmerling GJ, Neefjes JJ (1994) Trimming of TAP-translocated peptides in the endoplasmic reticulum and in the cytosol during recycling. J Exp Med 180:1591–1597
Rotem-Yehudar R, Winograd S, Sela S, Coligan JE, Ehrlich R (1994) Downregulation of peptide transporter genes in cell lines transformed with highly oncogenic adenovirus 12. J Exp Med 180:477–488
Rotem-Yehudar R, Groetrupp M, Soza A, Kloetzel PM, Ehrlich R (1996) LMP-associated proteolytic activities and TAP-dependent peptide transport for class I MHC molecules are suppressed in cell lines transformed by the highly oncogenic adenovirus 12. J Exp Med 183:499–514
Rowe M, Khanna R, Jacob CA, Argaet V, Kelly A, Powis S, Belich M, Croom-Carter D, Lee S, Burrows SR, Trowsdale J, Moss DJ, Rickinson AB (1995) Restoration of endogenous antigen processing in Burkitt's lymphoma cells by Epstein-Barr virus latent membrane protein-1: coordinate up-regulation of peptide transporters and HLA-class I antigen expression. Eur J Immunol 25:1374–1384
Ruiz-Cabello F, Klein E, Garrido F (1991) MHC antigens on human tumors. Immunol Letters 29:181–189
Salcedo M, Momburg F, Hämmerling GJ, Ljunggren HG (1994) Resistance to natural killer cell lysis conferred by TAP1/2 genes in human antigen-processing mutant cells. J Immunol 152:1702–1708
Sanda MG, Restifo NP, Walsh JC, Kawakami Y, Nelson WG, Pardoll DM, Simons JW (1995) Molecular characterization of defective antigen processing in human prostate cancer. J Natl Cancer Inst 87:280–285
Schrier PI, Bernards R, Vaessen RTMJ, Houweling A, van der Eb AJ (1983) Expression of class I MHC switched off by highly oncogenic adenovirus 12 in transformed rat cells. Nature 305:771–775
Schumacher TNM, Bruijn MLH, Vernie LN, Kast WM, Melief CJM, Neefjes JJ, Ploegh HL (1991) Peptide selection of MHC class I molecules. Nature 350: 703–706
Schumacher TNM, Kantesaria DV, Heemels MT, Ashton-Rickardt PG, Shepherd JC, Früh K, Young Y, Peterson PA, Tonegawa S, Ploegh HL (1994) Peptide length and sequence specificity of mouse TAP1/TAP2 translocator. J Exp Med 179:533–540
Seliger B, Höhne A, Knuth A, Bernhard H et al (1996a) Analysis of the major histocompatibility complex class I antigen presentation machinery in normal and malignant renal cells: evidence for deficiencies associated with transformation and progression. Cancer Res 56:1756–1760
Seliger B, Höhne A, Knuth A, Bernhard H, Ehring B, Tampé R, Huber C (1996b) Reduced membrane major histocompatibility complex class I density and stability in a subset of human renal cell carcinomas with low TAP and LMP expression. Clin Cancer Res 2:1427–1433
Shemesh J, Ehrlich R (1993) Aberrant biosynthesis and transport of class I major histocompatibility complex molecules in cells transformed with highly oncogenic human adenoviruses. J Biol Chem 268:15704–15711
Shemesh J, Rotem-Yeduhar R, Ehrlich R (1991) Transcriptional and posttranscriptional regulation of class I major histocompatibility complex genes following infection and transformation with human adenoviruses. J Virol 65:5544–5548
Shepherd JC, Schumacher TNM, Ashton-Rickardt PG, Imaeda S, Ploegh HL, Janeway CA Jr, Tonegawa S (1993) TAP1-dependent peptide translocation in vitro is ATP dependent and peptide selective. Cell 74:577–584
Spies T, DeMars RA (1991) Restored expression of the major histocompatibility class I molecules by gene transfer of a putative peptide transporter. Nature 351:323–324
Spies T, Bresnahan M, Bahram S, Arnold D, Blanck G, Mellins E, Pious D, DeMars R (1990) A gene in the human major histocompatibility complex class II region controlling the class I antigen presentation pathway. Nature 348:744–747

Suh WK, Cohen-Doyle M, Früh K, Wang, K, Peterson PA, Williams DB (1994) Interaction of MHC class I molecules with the transporter associated with antigen processing. Science 264:1322–1326

Tanaka K, Isselbacher A, Khoury G, Jay G (1985) Reversal of oncogenesis by the expression of a major histocompatibility complex class I gene. Science 228:26–33

Ting JPY, Baldwin AS (1993) Regulation of MHC gene expression. Curr Opin Immunol 5:8-16

Townsend A, Bodmer H (1989) Antigen recognition by class I-restricted T lymphocytes. Annu Rev Immunol 7:601–624

Townsend A, Öhlén C, Bastin J, Ljunggren HG, Foster L, Kärre K (1989) Association of class I major histocompatibility heavy and light chains induced by viral peptides. Nature 340:443–448

Trowsdale J, Hanson I, Mockridge I, Beck S, Townsend A, Kelly A (1990) Sequences encoded in the class II region of the MHC related to the "ABC" superfamily of transporters. Nature 348:741–744

Uebel S, Meyer TH, Kraas W, Kienle S, Jung G, Wiesmüller KH, Tampé R (1995) Requirements for peptide binding to the human transporter associated with antigen-processing revealed by peptide scans and complex peptide libraries. J Biol Chem 270:18512–18516

van Endert PM, Tampé R, Meyer TH, Tisch R, Bach JF, McDevitt HO (1994) A sequential model of peptide binding and transport by the transporters associated with antigen processing. Immunity 1:491–500

van Kaer L, Ashton-Rickardt PG, Ploegh HL, Tonegawa S (1992) TAP1 mutant mice are deficient in antigen presentation, surface class I molecules and $CD4^-CD8^+$ T cells. Cell 71:1205–1214

Wei ML, Cresswell P (1992) HLA-A2 molecules in an antigen processing mutant cell contain signal sequence derived peptides. Nature 356:443–446

Wölfel T, Klehmann E, Müller C, Schutt KH, Meyer zum Büschenfelde KH, Knuth A (1989) Lysis of melanoma cells by autologous cytolytic T cell clones: identification of human histocompatibility leukocyte antigen A2 as a restriction element for three different antigens. J Exp Med 170:797–810

Wölfel T, VanPel A, Brichard V, Schneider J, Seliger B, Meyer zum Büschenfelde KH, Boon T (1994) Two tyrosinase nonapeptides recognized on HLA-A2 melanomas by autologous cytolytic T lymphocytes. Eur J Immunol 24:759–764

Wright KL, White LC, Kelly A, Beck S, Trowsdale J, Ting JP-Y (1995) Coordinate regulation of the human TAP1 and LMP2 genes from a shared bidirectional promoter. J Exp Med 181:1459–1471

Yang Y, Früh K, Chambers J, Waters JB, Wu L, Spies T, Petersson PA (1992) Major histocompatibiliy complex (MHC)-encoded HAM2 is necessary for antigenic peptide loading onto class I MHC molecules. J Biol Chem 267:11669–11672

Yewdell JW, Bennink JR (1992) Cell biology of antigen processing and presentation to MHC class I molecule restricted T lymphocytes. Annu Rev Immunol 52:1–123

Zinkernagel RM, Doherty PC (1979) MHC restricted cytotoxic T cells: studies on the biological role of polymorphic major transplantation antigens determining T cell restriction specificity, function and responsiveness. Adv Immunol 27:51–177

Zweerink HJ, Gammon MC, Utz U, Sauma SY, Harrer T, Hawkins JC, Sirotina A, Hermes JD, Walker BD, Biddison WE (1993) Presentation of endogenous peptides to MHC class I restricted cytotoxic T lymphocytes in transport deletion mutant T2 cells. J Immunol 150:1763–1771

The Use of HLA Transgenic Mice in Identifying and Targeting Human Tumor Cell Antigens

L. A. SHERMAN, M. THEOBALD, AND J. LUSTGARTEN

Introduction

Identification of tumor-specific antigens remains an important challenge for tumor immunology. In recent years, significant progress towards this goal has been made by using the immune system of the tumor-bearing host to identify relevant tumor antigens. For example, examination of the specificity of tumor-infiltrating lymphocytes (TILs) has led to the identification of a series of melanoma specific antigens [1–4]. Although tissue-specific, these are of value due to their expression in tumors from different patients, thereby raising the possibility of a general immunotherapy or vaccine approach to stimulate the immune system.

However, it is restrictive to rely on the immune system of the tumor-bearing host to identify all potential tumor antigens. Indeed, many tumors express potentially antigenic epitopes; however, the tumor cells themselves may be poor stimulators [5]. This may often be due to low levels of expression of MHC molecules [6], or lack of expression of co-stimulatory molecules necessary for T-cell activation [7, 8]. Alternatively, the host may exhibit T-cell tolerance. For example, there are proteins such as p53 and Her-2neu that are known to be expressed at high levels in tumor cells from a broad variety of tumors and therefore are potential targets of immunotherapy. However, due to their expression at low levels in some types of normal cells, these proteins would also represent natural toleragens, thereby preventing immune responses. This is particularly true of molecules expressed in the thymus, as such expression would lead to the deletion of potentially autoreactive T cells [9].

To override problems related to poor immunogenicity or deficiencies in the T cell repertoire, we have turned to HLA transgenic mice as an alternative means of identifying tumor antigens. In addition to providing a means to perform in vivo immunization to identify antigens, they also have the additional advantage that due to species differences in protein sequence, mice may not be tolerant of human proteins that could be tumor associated antigens.

Symposium in Immunology VI
Eibl/Huber/Peter/Wahn (Eds.)

HLA Transgenic Mice

A major barrier to recognition and utilization of human class I HLA antigens by mouse T cells is the inability of murine CD8 to interact with human class I molecules [10–12]. Transgenic mice that express A2.1 demonstrate a weak A2.1-restricted response to viral antigens [13, 14]. Several different strategies have been used successfully to overcome this barrier in order to develop murine models capable of developing more vigorous HLA-restricted T-cell responses. Changes can be made within portions of the HLA molecule that affect CD8 interaction without affecting T cell receptor (TCR) recognition, thus allowing murine CD8 T cells to interact with the human class I HLA antigen. This was the rationale for constructing a chimeric molecule, HLA-A2.1/K^b, in which the $\alpha1$ and $\alpha2$ domains are of A2.1 origin and the $\alpha3$ domain that interacts with CD8 is derived from the K^b molecule [10, 15]. When immunized with influenza, such mice develop an influenza-specific cytotoxic T-lymphocyte (CTL) response with CTLs restricted to the A2/K^b transgene. Importantly, as demonstrated for several different viral and tumor antigens, these T cells recognize the same peptide antigens that are immunogenic in A2.1 humans. Thus, HLA A2/K^b transgenic mice infected with influenza respond to the same dominant peptide antigen from the viral matrix protein that is recognized in A2.1 positive humans [15]. This indicates that the processing and presentation machinery in mouse and human cells is sufficiently similar to present the same antigens. Furthermore, the TCR repertoire in man and mouse is also sufficiently diverse to respond to these same peptide-MHC combinations. In a recent study in which 38 different peptides that bind A2. 1 were used to compare the ability of A2/K^b transgenic mice and human peripheral blood leukocytes (PBL) to respond to peptide antigens, it was found that there was 71% correlation overall [16]. Interestingly, among the peptides that bound A2.1 with highest affinity, this correlation was 85%. Accordingly, HLA transgenic mice represent an important tool in identifying antigens under experimental conditions that require in vivo immunization.

An alternative strategy that leads to a vigorous A2.1-restricted response is to produce a double transgenic mouse that expresses both A2.1 and the human CD8 molecule [14, 17]. As demonstrated in Fig. 1 this also leads to an A2.1-restricted influenza response comparable to that obtained in the A2/K^b transgenic mouse. An advantage of deriving T cells that express human CD8 is their ability to interact with human target cells that express the intact A2.1 molecule rather than A2/K^b.

Finally, it should be considered that although it can be difficult to obtain an A2.1-restricted response in mice expressing the intact A2.1 molecule, those CTLs that are obtained express TCRs with unusually high affinity for the relevant peptide-A2.1 complex. Unlike normal T-cell responses in which both CD8 and TCR contribute to the avidity of interaction that ultimately leads to

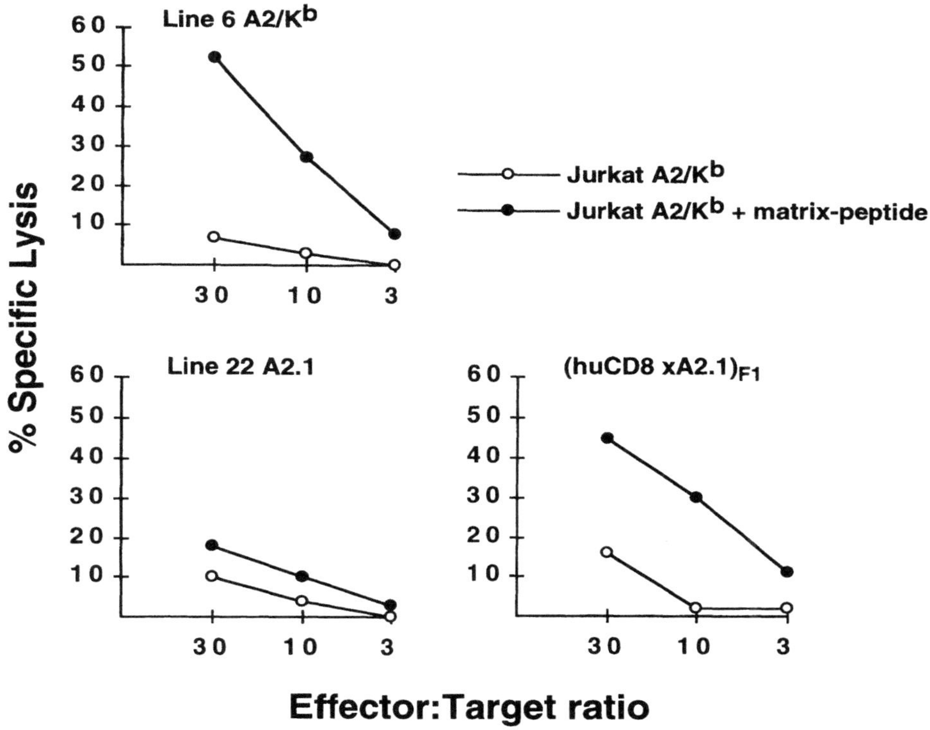

Fig. 1. Comparison of transgenic mice with respect to their A2.1-restricted response to influenza. The indicated type of transgenic mouse was immunized with influenza virus in vivo and CTL cultures established as previously described [14]

stimulation, T cells from A2.1 transgenic mice have been stimulated without the benefit of CD8 interaction and therefore only those with unusually high TCR affinity are successfully activated [14, 18].

Identification of A2-restricted Peptides from p53

p53 normally functions within the nucleus as a tumor suppressor gene, preventing division by cells with mutated or damaged DNA [19–22]. This normal function is critical in preventing cells from propagating mutations. However, once p53 is itself mutated, the altered protein no longer serves as a tumor suppressor and it accumulates at high levels in the cytoplasm. Due to its high level of expression in many different types of tumor cells, p53 represents an excellent candidate for a tumor associated antigen. However, it is likely that normal levels of expression of p53 in the thymus is sufficient to lead to tolerance within the T-cell compartment of epitopes representing wild type sequence. Nevertheless, human and mouse p53 are sufficiently different to anticipate immune recognition in HLA transgenic mice immunized with human p53. Our goal was to use these mice to identify peptides from human p53 that were presented in association with A2.1 and to determine which of these peptides was immunogenic [18].

The approach we took to identify p53 peptides recognized by CD8+ T cells from HLA transgenic mice in association with HLA-A2.1 was to first identify peptides from the human p53 protein that exhibit the characteristic motif necessary for binding to A2.1 (L, M, I, V, A, or T at position 2 and V, L, I, A, M, T, S, or Q at the COOH-terminus). A competition assay was used to determine if the synthesized peptides actually bound A2.1. Peptides capable of blocking the binding of the influenza matrix peptide to A2.1, as assessed by inhibition of lysis by matrix-peptide specific CTLs, were judged capable of binding A2.1 and further analyzed for their ability to stimulate a CTL response in HLA transgenic mice. Mice were immunized subcutaneously at the base of the tail with a mixture of 100 μg of the p53 peptide and 120 μg of a peptide known to be immunogenic for CD4 helper T cells, residues 128–140 of the hepatitis B virus core protein, both emulsified in incomplete Freund's adjuvant. After 10 days, the spleen was removed and the cells restimulated in vitro using antigen-presenting cells pulsed with the same p53 peptide used for in vivo priming. This type of protocol led to the identification of four peptides that could elicit an A2.1-restricted CTL response.

In order to determine which, if any, of these p53 peptides were endogenously processed and presented on the cell surface with A2.1 in human cells that express p53, it was necessary to determine if CTLs which were originally identified on the basis of lysis of peptide-pulsed cells could also recognize human tumor cells. Only two of the four peptide-specific CTL populations were able to lyse cells that endogenously expressed p53 and were A2.1-positive. These two CTL populations were further tested for their ability to kill a large panel of human tumor cells. Many of the A2+ tumors, representing a variety of tissue types, were killed by p53-specific CTLs. It should be noted that efficient killing did not occur unless the tumor was precultured for 24 h in media containing both γ-interferon and tumor necrosis factor-α. Such preincubation increases the expression of MHC–peptide complexes, adhesion molecules, and Fas [23, 24]. Depending upon the particular type of tumor, any or all of these changes could contribute to enhanced susceptibility of lysis, and it was necessary to observe lysis of these same tumors by allospecific CTL. Another important feature of these data is that non-transformed cells, as represented by dendritic cells or lymphoblasts, were not lysed. This suggests that normal cells undergoing replication may not be susceptible to lysis by p53-specific CTLs due to the relatively low levels of p53 expressed by normal cells.

It is of interest to compare these results with those of other laboratories that have used human PBLs to obtain responses to p53 peptides. Several of the peptides identified as immunogenic in the A2/K^b mice were also identified in such cultures and found to be able to stimulate a peptide-specifc, A2.1-restricted response by human PBLs [25–27]. The significant difference is that whereas the murine CTLs were able to lyse human tumor cells, this has not been reported for p53-peptide-specific human PBLs. It is possible that this reflects the low avidity of the human p53-specific CTLs that survived self-tolerance.

Development of Her-2neu-Specific CTLs

Another tumor associated protein that is expressed at high levels in a broad range of tumors is Her-2neu [28]. As is the case with p53, it is expressed at low levels in some normal tissues; however, the differential level of expression in normal and transformed cells potentially provides a window of opportunity for CTL intervention [29, 30]. Using the same strategy described above to identify immunogenic peptides from p53, we identified two peptides from Her-2neu that were presented by A2.1+, Her-2neu-expressing human tumors (Lustgarten and Sherman, manuscript in preparation). The specificity of these CTLs was ascertained by their ability to lyse human tumor cells that were both A2.1+ and Her-2neu+, but not cells negative for either protein. As was true with p53-specific CTL, optimal lysis required preincubation of tumor cells in cytokines. Interestingly, one of the peptides identified in this study was also identified by others studying the specificity of human TILs [23].

In vivo Destruction of Tumors Using Her-2neu-Specific CTLs

The experiments described above demonstrate the ability of p53- and Her-2neu-specific CTLs to kill a broad range of tumors in vitro. In order to determine if the CTLs are capable of rejecting tumors in vivo, a model was used in which A2.1+ human tumor cells expressing high levels of Her-2neu were propagated in SCID mice. Two different human tumor cell lines were tested in such studies, the breast adenocarcinoma cell line, MDA.MB.231 and the non-small cell carcinoma NCI-H1355. In both cases, the presence of Her-2neu-specific CTLs succeeded in significantly slowing down the rate of tumor cell growth. In the case of NCI-H1355, the continuous administration of interleukin-2 was also found to be necessary (Lustgarten and Sherman, unpublished observation).

Transfer of TCR Genes with Tumor Specificity

In cases in which the T-cell repertoire of the tumor-bearing host contains quiescent tumor-specific T cells, the best approach for immunotherapy may be a strategy that leads to a more efficient activation of these cells, such as the development of vaccines and adjuvants to boost the immune response to tumor-specific antigens. Also in this category are approaches that strive to augment the immunogenicity of the tumor through expression of appropriate co-stimulatory molecules. However, in other situations in which the host's immune system is devoid of such precursors, an alternative strategy would be one in which the genes for tumor specific TCRs are transferred to the patient's T cells. In the past few years there have been several reports in which TCR genes have been modified and used to transfer specificity [31–33]. The most efficient approach is to attach to the TCR an intracellular domain that enables direct signal transduction. This overrides the necessity of relying upon appropriate interaction with the endogenous TCR complex in order to transduce a stimulatory signal, and has been successfully achieved by using the intracellular portion of CD3ε or TCRζ connected to the TCR molecule [32, 33]. The extracellular domains can consist of either a single chain or double chain molecule. We have produced such molecules using the TCRs from a Her-2neu-specific CTL clone that recognized peptide and used the constructs to transfect a T-cell hybridoma (27 J) that does not express an endogenous TCR molecule. When incubated with HLA-A2.1+ antigen-presenting cells and the appropriate peptide, the hybridoma responds specifically to produce IL-2 (Lustgarten and Sherman, manuscript in preparation). In the future, this type of approach could be used to transfer specificity for tumor antigens to normal PBLs of the tumor-bearing patient.

References

1. van der Bruggen P, Traversari C, Chomez P, Lurquin C, De Plaen E, Van den Eynde B, Knuth A, Boon T (1991) A gene encoding an antigen recognized by cytolytic T lymphocytes on a human melanoma. Science 254:1643–1647
2. Bakker ABH, Schreurs MWJ, Boer AJD, Kawakami Y, Rosenberg SA, Adema GJ, Figdor CG (1994) Melanocyte lineage-specific antigen gp100 is recognized by melanoma-derived tumor-infiltrating lymphocytes. J Exp Med 179:1005–1009
3. Brichard V, Van Pel A, Wölfel T, Wolfel C, De Plaen E, Lethé B, Coulie P, Boon T (1993) The tyrosinase gene codes for an antigen recognized by autologous cytolytic T lymphocytes on HLA-A2 melanomas. J Exp Med 178:489–495
4. Kawakami Y, Eliyahu S, Delgado CH, Robbins PF, Rivoltini L, Topalian SL, Miki T, Rosenberg SA (1994) Cloning of the gene coding for a shared human melanoma antigen recognized by autologous T cells infiltrating into tumor. Proc Natl Acad Sci USA 91:3515–3519
5. Boon T, Cerottini JC, Van den Eynde B, van der Bruggen P, Van Pel A (1994) Tumor antigens recognized by T lymphocytes. Annu Rev Immunol 12:337–365

6. Gansbacher B, Bannerji R, Daniels B, Zier K, Cronin K, Gilboa E (1990) Retroviral vector-mediated gamma-interferon gene transfer into tumor cells generates potent and long lasting anti-tumor immunity. Cancer Res 50:7820–7825
7. Chen L, Ashe S, Brady W, Hellström I, Ledbetter J, McGowan P, Linsley P (1992) Costimulation of antitumor immunity by the B7 counterreceptor for the T lymphocyte molecules CD28 and CLTA4. Cell 71:1093–1102
8. Townsend S, Allison J (1993) Tumor rejection after direct costimulation of CD8+ T cells by B7-transfected melanoma cells. Science 259:368–370
9. Rogel A, Popliker M, Webb CG, Oren M (1985) p53 cellular tumor antigen: analysis of mRNA levels in normal adult tissues, embryos, and tumors. Mol Cell Biol 5:2851–2855
10. Irwin MJ, Heath WR, Sherman LA (1989) Species-restricted interactions between CD8 and the α3 domain of class I influence the magnitude of the xenogenic response. J Exp Med 170:1091–1101
11. Samberg NL, Scarlett EC, Stauss HJ (1989) The α3 domain of major histocompatibility complex class I molecules play a critical role in cytotoxic T lymphyocyte stimulation. Eur J Immunol 19:2349
12. Kalinke U, Arnold B, Hammerling GJ (1990) Strong xenogenic HLA response in transgenic mice after introducing an α3 domain into HLA-B27. Nature 348:642
13. Man S, Ridge JP, Engelhard VH (1994) Diversity and dominance among TCR recognizing HLA-A2.1+ influenza matrix peptide in human MHC class I transgenic mice. J Immunol 153:4458–4467
14. Sherman LA, Hesse SV, Irwin MJ, Face DL, Peterson P (1992) Selecting T cell receptors with high affinity for self-MHC by decreasing the contribution of CD8. Science 258:815–818
15. Vitiello A, Marchesini D, Furze J, Sherman LA, Chestnut RW (1991) Analysis of the HLA-restricted influenza-specific CTL response in transgenic mice carrying a chimeric human-mouse class I MHC molecule. J Exp Med 173:1007–1015
16. Wentworth PA, Vitiello A, Sidney J, Keogh E, Chesnut RW, Grey H, Sette A (1996) Differences and similarities in the A2.1-restricted cytotoxic T cell repertoire in humans and human leukocyte antigen-transgenic mice. Eur J Immunol 26:97–101
17. LaFace DM, Vestberg M, Yang Y, Srivastava R, DiSanto J, Flomenberg N, Brown S, Sherman LA, Peterson PA (1995) Human CD8 coreceptor regulation of HLA recognition by murine T cells. J Exp Med 182:1315
18. Theobald M, Biggs J, Dittmer D, Levine AJ, Sherman LA (1995) Targeting p53 as a general tumor antigen. Proc Natl Acad Sci USA 92:11993–11997
19. Levine AJ, Momand J, Finlay CA (1991) The p53 tumor suppressor gene. Nature 351:453–456
20. Hollstein M, Sidransky D, Vogelstein B, Harris CC (1991) p53 mutations in human cancers. Science 253:49–53
21. Hartwell L (1992) Defects in a cell cycle checkpoint may be responsible for the genomic instability of cancer cells. (Review) Cell 71:543–546
22. Yonish-Rouach E, Resnitzky D, Lotem J, Sachs L, Kimchi A, Oren M (1991) Wild-type p53 induces apoptosis of myeloid leukaemic cells that is inhibited by interleukin-6. Nature 352:345–347
23. Fisk B, Blevins TL, Wharton JT, Ioannides CG (1995) Identification of an immunodominant peptide of HER-2/neu proto-oncogene recognized by ovarian tumor-specific cytotoxic T lymphocyte lines. J Exp Med 181:2109–2117
24. Fady C, Gardner A, Gera JF, Lichtenstein A (1993) Interferon-gamma-induced increased sensitivity of HER2/neu-overexpressing tumor cells to lymphokine-activated killer cell lysis: importance of ICAM-1 in binding and post-binding events. Cancer Immunol Immunother 37:329–336

25. Houbiers JGA, Nijman HW, van der Burg SH, Drijfhout JW, Kenemans P, van de Velde CJ, Brand A, Momburg F, Kast WM, Melief CJ (1993) In vitro induction of human cytotoxic T lymphocyte responses against peptides of mutant and wild-type p53. Eur J Immunol 23:2072–2077
26. Nijman HW, Houbiers JG, van der Burg SH, Vierboom MP, Kenemans P, Kast WM, Melief CJ (1993) Characterization of cytotoxic T lymphocyte epitopes of a self-protein, p53, and a non-self-protein, influenza matrix: relationship between major histocompatibility complex peptide binding affinity and immune responsiveness to peptides. J Immunother 14:121–126
27. Nijman HW, van der Burg SH, Vierboom MP, Houbiers JG, Kast WM, Melief CJ (1994) p53, a potential target for tumor-directed T cells. Immunol Lett 40:171–178
28. Slamon DJ, Godolphin W, Jones LA, Holt JA, Wong SG, Keith DE, Levin WJ, Stuart SG, Udove J, Ullrich A, Press MF (1989) Studies of the Her-2/neu proto-oncogene in human breast and ovarian cancer. Science 244:707
29. Natali PG, Nicotra MR, Bigotti A, Venturo I, Slamon DJ, Fendly BM, Ullrich A (1990) Expression of the p185 encoded by HER2 oncogene in normal and transformed human tissues. Int J Cancer 45:457–461
30. Press MF, Cordon-Cardo C, Slamon DJ (1990) Expression of the HER-2/neu proto-oncogene in normal human adult and fetal tissues. Oncogene 5:953–962
31. Novonty J, Ganju RK, Smiley ST, Husseym RE, Luther MA, Rency MA, Silciano RF, Reinherz EL (1991) A soluble single chain T cell receptor fragment endowed with antigen combining properties. Proc Natl Acad Sci USA 88:8646
32. Brocker T, Peter A, Traunecker A, Karjalainen K (1993) New simplified molecular design for functional T cell receptor. Eur J Immunol 23:1435–1439
33. Chung S, Wucherpfennig KW, Friedman SM, Hafler DA, Strominger JL (1994) Functional three-domain single-chain T-cell receptors. Proc Natl Acad Sci USA 91:12654–12658

CD95-Associating Signaling Molecules

M. E. Peter

Introduction

In recent years apoptosis has attracted more and more attention. In immunology it has become especially popular since it plays an important role in the development and maturation of normal T and B lymphocytes and in lymphoid malignancies. In the normal lymphoid system, apoptosis occurs in primary lymphoid organs such as the bone marrow, liver, and thymus, and is used to eliminate useless precursor cells with nonrearranged or aberrantly rearranged, nonfunctional receptors . Whether lymphocytes die by apoptosis or survive is controlled by various genes and their products. In principle, genes relevant for apoptosis might code for death or survival ligands and their receptors, or a cascade of signaling molecules. Such signaling molecules might be connected to second messengers and bridge membrane events to transcription factors and gene expression. Gene products might then either stimulate or block apoptosis.

Genes directly implicated in lymphoid apoptosis are *p53*, c-*myc*, *nur-77*, *pim*-1, several members of the *bcl*-2 family, and the gene for CD95 (APO-1/Fas; for a review see Krammer et al. 1994a). CD95 transduces an apoptotic signal in a variety of different tissues (for a review see Krammer et al. 1994b). CD95 belongs to the NGF/TNF-receptor superfamily, members of which need to be trimerized by specific protein ligands in order to generate a signal. Recently, progress has been made in the understanding of the proximal signal transduction mechanism of CD95. The cloning of genes encoding numerous proteins that interact with CD95 and other members of this receptor family and the in vivo identification of several proteins that associate with CD95 in a ligand-dependent fashion opens the way to delineate the death pathway and to explain crosstalk among these receptors at the molecularlevel.

Symposium in Immunology VI
Eibl/Huber/Peter/Wahn (Eds.)

The CD95 receptor

The role of CD95 and its ligand

CD95 is a type I transmembrane receptor of approximately 52 kDa that is heavily sialylated (Peter et al. 1995). It belongs to the nerve growth factor/tumor necrosis factor (NGF/TNF) receptor superfamily (NGF-R, TNF-R1, TNF-R2, CD27, CD30, CD40, 4-1BB, OX40; for a review see Smith et al. 1994) characterized by cysteine-rich extracellular domains. Apoptosis via the CD95 receptor can be triggered by agonistic antibodies such as anti-APO-1 and by the natural ligand of the receptor. The CD95 ligand (CD95L) was shown to be a TNF-related type II transmembrane molecule (members of the ligand family: TNF, LT, LTβ, CD27L, CD30L, CD40L, and TRAIL). Although expressed in a variety of tissues and cell lines, the predominant physiologic role of CD95 may be in the regulation of the immune system. This is exemplified by the phenotype of MRL/*lpr* mice showing a strongly reduced CD95 expression (Mariani et al. 1994). *lpr* mice develop lymphadenopathy and splenomegaly and generate large quantities of autoantibodies. The primary cause of this fatal syndrome in mice is the inability to delete peripheral, autoreactive lymphocytes by the CD95 system (Singer et al. 1994).

The cytoplasmic region of human CD95 (in total, 325 amino acids) consists of 145 amino acids and does not contain any known consensus sequences for enzymatic functions or binding sites for any known signaling molecules. It has homology to TNF-R1 which has also been shown to transduce a cytotoxic signal (Tartaglia et al. 1991). Itoh and Nagata defined an area of 65 amino acids, the "death domain", present in both CD95 and TNF-R1 and responsible for promoting the death signal (Itoh and Nagata 1993). This domain was characterized in detail in the TNF-R1 as an 80 amino acid domain essential for triggering cell death (Tartaglia et al. 1993). The importance of the death domain for CD95 signaling is also demonstrated by the *lpr*^{Cg} mice. These mice have a phenotype similar to *lpr* mice. However they carry a point mutation located within the death domain of CD95 resulting in signaling deficiency (Watanabe-Fukunaga et al. 1992).

CD95-Associated Molecules and the CD95 Death-inducing Signaling Complex

Recently, we have shown that CD95 signaling does not involve "classic" signaling pathways such as activation of protein tyrosine kinases (Schraven and Peter 1995; for a review see Peter at al. 1996). CD95 signaling seems to involve a set of unique and novel signaling molecules. During the last year a number of new signaling molecules were identified that associate with death-domain-containing receptors such as CD95. In addition, a 65 amino acid death-domain-containing protein called reaper was found to be associated with apoptosis in *Drosophila* (White et al. 1994; Golstein 1995). This underlines the importance of the death domain protein structure for apoptosis.

However, a number of proteins not involved in apoptosis that also contain a death domain were recently discovered by an intensive search of data bases for sequences with homology to the death domain (Feinstein et al. 1995; Hofmann and Tschopp 1995). It is becoming apparent that the death domain is a specific protein structure that facilitates protein aggregation and in some cases apoptosis. How protein aggregation can induce cell death is unclear.

Last year, the yeast two-hybrid system allowed identification of a number of proteins binding to CD95:

1. FAP-1 is a protein tyrosine phosphatase that associates with the negative regulatory domain of the receptor (the C-terminal 15 amino acids; Sato et al. 1995a). FAP-1 is unlikely to be directly involved in CD95 signaling since it is not expressed in Jurkat T cells, which are highly CD95-sensitive. However, overexpression of FAP-1 rendered Jurkat T cells resistant to anti-CD95-induced apoptosis.
2. RIP associates with CD95 in yeast and when overexpressed causes apoptosis in transfected cells (Stanger et al. 1995). The N-terminus of RIP contains a kinase domain; the C-terminal death domain of RIP associates with CD95 in the yeast two-hybrid system.
3. FADD/MORT1 was independently cloned by two different groups (Chinnaiyan et al. 1995; Boldin et al. 1995). It contains a death domain and induces apoptosis when overexpressed in different cells. Analysis of various deletion mutants of FADD/MORT1 demonstrated that the C-terminal death domain is responsible for association with CD95, while the N-terminus is required for self-association and to trigger apoptosis. Therefore, the death domain might be a CD95 association domain rather than a killing domain. This excludes the possibility that FADD/MORT1 causes apoptosis by simply aggregating intracellular CD95 since the N-terminus is unable to bind the receptor. FADD/MORT1 mRNA is expressed in all tissues and at all developmental stages tested (Chinnaiyan et al. 1995). Using an affinity-purified rabbit anti-FADD antibody, FADD/MORT1 protein was immunoblotted in all cells tested including Jurkat, HPB-All, HUT78, H9, peripheral T cells, BJAB, BL-60, K50, SKW6.4, Boe^R, 293T, L929, HepG2, MCF7, COLO205, and HT29 (Kischkel et al. 1995 and unpublished data). The ubiquitous expression of FADD/MORT1 suggests that it may play a key role in signaling cell death.

The in vitro association of RIP and FADD/MORT1 with CD95 suggested that these molecules are biologically important (Boldin et al. 1995; Chinnaiyan et al. 1995; Stanger et al. 1995). The N-terminus of FADD/MORT1 was shown to be both essential and sufficient to induce apoptosis in transfected cells (Chinnaiyan et al. 1995) and RIP contains a putative N-terminal kinase domain (Stanger et al. 1995). Both proteins therefore represent putative apoptosis effector molecules.

Cross-linking of CD95 by the IgG3 anti-APO-1 antibody initiated an in vivo association of receptors with four proteins designated CAP1–4 for cytotoxicity-dependent APO-1-associated proteins (Kischkel et al. 1995). Recruitment of these proteins occurred instantly and was dependent on CD95 oligomerization. CAP1 and CAP2 were identified as serine phosphorylated FADD/MORT1. The identity of the other CAP proteins, CAP3 and CAP4, remains to be determined. The associating CAP proteins along with the oligomerized CD95 have been termed the CD95 death-inducing signaling complex (DISC).

Of the three proteins found with the two-hybrid system to associate with CD95 so far only FADD/MORT1 could be established as a protein that binds in vivo to CD95 in a ligand-dependent fashion. FADD/MORT1 fulfills all criteria for being the main CD95 death transducing molecule. Apoptosis induced by CD95 and by FADD overexpression share certain features: CD95-mediated apoptosis is completely inhibited by the viral serpin inhibitor CrmA, suggesting that interleukin-1β converting enzyme (ICE)-like proteases are part of the CD95 cell death pathway (Tewari and Dixit 1995; Enari et al. 1995; Los et al. 1995). Apoptosis induced by overexpression of FADD/MORT1 is also CrmA-inhibitable (Chinnaiyan et al. 1996). In addition, both CD95-mediated and FADD/MORTl-induced cell death is inhibited by bcl-2, bcl-x_L, and the baculovirus protein p35 (Jaattela et al. 1995; Itoh et al. 1993; Beidler et al. 1995; Chinnaiyan et al. 1996) suggesting that a similar cell death program is triggered by CD95 and FADD/MORT1.

In addition, the CD95 signaling cascade involves cleavage of poly(ADP-ribose) polymerase (PARP) and the 70-kDa small nuclear ribonucleoprotein (snRP) U1–70 (Tewari et al. 1995a; Tewari et al. 1995b). Overexpression of FADD/MORT1 also causes PARP and U1–70 cleavage suggesting activation of the same proteases as upon CD95 triggering (Chinnaiyan et al. 1996).

As previously reported, a deletion mutant of FADD/MORT1 that includes the death domain failed to induce apoptosis (NFD-4 in Chinnaiyan et al. 1995). This version of FADD/MORT1 acted as a dominant negative (DN) inhibitor of CD95 signaling and was termed FADD-DN (Chinnaiyan et al. 1996). Expression of FADD-DN abolished the activity of various indicators of CD95 signal transduction including Yama and ceramide. Most importantly, it prevented the induction of apoptosis. In transfected cells FADD-DN associated with the receptor in a ligand-dependent fashion displacing the other endogenous CAP and thus, a complete DISC failed to form and the death signal was abrogated. In addition, the lack of CAP3 and CAP4 binding to the DISC suggests that the N-terminus of FADD/MORT1 is required for their recruitment.

Taken together, these results suggest that FADD/MORT1 is the essential component of the DISC for three reasons (1) Overexpression of FADD/MORT1 mimics all features of the CD95 cell death pathway; (2) A number of CD95-sensitive tissues have been tested and FADD/MORT1 is always a prominent component of the DISC (unpublished data); and (3) FADD-DN abrogates CD95 signaling and binds the receptor in a ligand-dependent fashion by physically preventing wildtype FADD from forming a CD95 DISC.

Proteins that Associate with other Members of the TNF-R Superfamily

All other members of the TNF-R family are also believed to be trimerized by their respective ligands (Smith et al. 1994). The signal transduction pathways have long been enigmatic. As in CD95 there are no identifiable catalytic motifs (e.g., kinases or phosphatases) in the cytoplasmic domains of these cell surface receptors. Instead, signal transduction is accomplished via association with an emerging class of novel and diverse signaling molecules. Candidate signal transducers first identified were TRAF1 and TRAF2 which bind to TNF-R2 (Rothe et al. 1994). They both contain a C terminal TNF receptor associated factor (TRAF) domain and form homo- and heterodimers. TRAF2 mediates binding of TRAF1 to the C-terminal half of TNF-R2. Soon after TRAF1 and TRAF2 were cloned, a related molecule, TRAF3/CD40bp/CRAF1/LAP1/CAP-1 was identified and shown to interact with CD40 (Rothe et al. 1995; Hu et al. 1994; Cheng et al. 1995; Mosialos et al. 1995; Sato et al. 1995b).

TRADD has been shown to associate with TNF-R1. It seems to be responsible for both NF-κB activation and induction of apoptosis which is CrmA-inhibitable (Hsu et al. 1995). In contrast to CD95-associated FADD/MORT1, it was found that the death domain (amino acids 195–305) alone of TRADD could interact with TNF-R1 **and** signal effectively. Since the TRADD death domain by itself is signaling competent, the question arises whether this domain can both associate with its receptor **and** couple with downstream signaling effector molecules. Recently, it was shown that the N-terminal TRADD domain interacts with TRAF2 resulting in NF-κB activation and the C-terminal domain binds death domain proteins such as FADD or TNF-R1 leading to apoptosis (Hsu et al. 1996).

Conclusion

The discovery of a family of novel signaling molecules that interact with members of the TNF-R family facilitates the investigation of the signaling pathways of these receptors. CD95 signaling is most complex. So far, the greatest number of interacting proteins were found to interact with the death domain of CD95. Although it has been established that FADD/MORT1 is the most important molecule in CD95 signaling, many important questions remain unresolved: firstly, what is the function of the other DISC components, CAP3 and CAP4, and of the other identified proteins, RIP and FAP-1? Secondly, how are the various levels in the apoptosis pathway such as DISC formation, activation of sphingomyelinases, and activation of ICE-like proteases linked to each other. Thirdly, are some of these putative molecules that are ubiquitously expressed, utilized in other cell death pathways, receptor-mediated or otherwise? All of these questions will have to be addressed in the future in order to understand the CD95 pathway. Only a good knowledge of this pathway will eventually result in the generation of agents to interfere with this kind of apoptosis. This will be crucial for the treatment of diseases where apoptosis is dysregulated such as AIDS or cancer.

References

Beidler DR, Tewari M, Friesen PD, Poirier G, Dixit VM (1995) The baculovirus p35 protein inhibits Fas- and tumor necrosis factor-induced apoptosis. J Biol Chem 270:16526–16528

Boldin MP, Varfolomeev EE, Pancer Z, Mett IL, Camonis JH, Wallach D (1995) A novel protein that interacts with the death domain of Fas/APOl contains a sequence motif related to the death domain. J Biol Chem 270:7795–7798

Cheng G, Cleary AM, Ye ZS, Hong DI, Lederman S, Baltimore D (1995) Involvement of CRAF1, a relative of TRAF, in CD40 signaling. Science 267:1494–1498

Chinnaiyan AM, O'Rourke K, Tewari M, Dixit VM (1995) FADD, a novel death domain-containing protein interacts with the death domain of Fas and initiates apoptosis. Cell 81:505–512

Chinnaiyan AM, Tepper CG, Seldin MF, O'Rourke K, Lou L, Kischkel FC, Hellbardt S, Krammer PH, Peter ME, Dixit VM (1996) FADD/MORT1 is a common mediator of Fas/APO-1- and tumor necrosis factor-induced apoptosis. J Biol Chem (In press)

Enari M, Hug H, Nagata S (1995) Involvement of an ICE-like protease in Fas-mediated apoptosis. Nature 375:78–81

Feinstein E, Kimchi A, Wallach D, Boldin M, Varfolomeev E (1995) The death domain: a module shared by proteins with diverse cellular functions. Trends Biochem Sci 20:342–344

Golstein P, Marguet D, Depraetere V (1995) Homology between reaper and the cell death domains of Fas and TNFR1. Cell 81:185–186

Hofmann K, Tschopp J (1995) The death domain motif in Fas(Apo-1) and TNF receptor is present in proteins involved in apoptosis and axonal guidance. FEBS Lett 371:321–323

Hsu H, Xiong J, Goeddel DV (1995) The TNF receptor 1-associated protein TRADD signals cell death and NF-κB activation. Cell 81:495–504

Hsu H, Shu H-B, Pan M-G, Goeddel DV (1996) TRADD–TRAF2 and TRADD–FADD interactions define two distinct TNF receptor 1 signal transduction pathways. Cell 84:299–308

Hu HM, O'Rouke K, Boguski MS, Dixit VM (1994) A novel RING finger protein interacts with the cytoplasmic domain of CD40. J Biol Chem 269:30069–30072

Itoh N, Nagata S (1993) A novel protein domain required for apoptosis. Mutational analysis of human Fas antigen. J Biol Chem 268:10932–10937

Itoh N, Tsujimoto Y, Nagata S (1993) Effect of bcl-2 on Fas antigen-mediated cell death. J Immunol 151:621–627

Jaattela M, Benedict M, Tewari M, Shayman JA, Dixit VM (1995) Bcl-x and Bcl-2 inhibit TNF and Fas-induced apoptosis and activation of phospholipase A2 in breast carcinoma cells. Oncogene 10:2297–2305

Kischkel FC, Hellbardt S, Behrmann I, Germer M, Pawlita M, Krammer PH, Peter ME (1995) Cytotoxicity-dependent APO-1(Fas/CD95)-associated proteins form a death-inducing signalling complex (DISC) with the receptor. EMBO J 14:5579–5588

Krammer PH, Behrmann I, Daniel P, Dhein J, Debatin K-M (1994a) Regulation of apoptosis in the immune system. Curr Op in Immunol 6:279–289

Krammer PH, Dhein J, Walczak H, Behrmann I, Mariani S, Matiba B, Fath M, Daniel PT, Knipping E, Westendorp MO, Stricker K, Bäumler C, Hellbardt S, Germer M, Peter ME, Debatin K-M (1994b) The role of APO-1-mediated apoptosis in the immune system. Immunol Rev 142:175–191

Los M, van de Craen M, Penning L, Schenk H, Westendorp M, Bäuerle P, Dröge W, Krammer PH, Fiers W, Schulze-Osthoff K (1995) Requirement of an ICE/CED-3 protease for Fas/APO-1-mediated apoptosis. Nature 375:81–83

Mariani SM, Matiba B, Armandola EA, Krammer PH (1994) The APO-1/Fas (CD95) receptor is expressed in homozygous MRL/lpr mice. Eur J Immunol 24:3119–3123

Mosialos G, Birkenbach M, Yalamanchili R, VanArdale T, Ware C, Kieff E (1995) The Epstein-Barr virus transforming protein LMP1 engages signaling proteins for the tumor necrosis factor receptor family. Cell 80:389–399

Peter ME, Hellbardt S, Schwartz-Albiez R, Westendorp MO, Walczak H, Moldenhauer G, Grell M, Krammer PH (1995) Cell surface sialylation plays a role in modulating sensitivity towards APO-1-mediated apoptotic cell death. Cell Death Differ 2:163–171

Peter ME, Kischkel FC, Hellbardt S, Chinnaiyan AM, Krammer PH, Dixit VM (1996). CD95(APO-1/Fas)-associating signaling proteins. Cell Death Differ 3:171–176

Rothe M, Wong SC, Henzel WJ, Goeddel DV (1994) A novel family of putative signal transducers associated with the cytoplasmic domain of the 75 kDa tumor necrosis factor receptor. Cell 78:681–692

Rothe M, Sarma V, Dixit M, Goeddel DV (1995) TRAF2-mediated activation of NF-κB by TNF receptor 2 and CD40. Science 269:1424–1427

Sato T, Irie S, Kitada S, Reed JC (1995a) FAP-1: a protein tyrosine phosphatase that associates with Fas. Science 268:411–413

Sato T, Irie S, Reed JC (1995b) A novel member of the TRAF family of putative signal transducing proteins binds to the cytosolic domain of CD40. FEBS Lett 358:113–118

Schraven B, Peter ME (1995) APO-1(CD95)-mediated apoptosis in Jurkat cells does not involve src kinases or CD45. FEBS Lett 368:491–494

Singer GG, Carrera AC, Marshak-Rothstein A, Martinez C, Abbas AK (1994) Apoptosis, Fas and systemic autoimmunity: the MRL-lpr/lpr model. Curr Opin Immunol 6:913–920

Smith CA, Farrah T, Goodwin RG (1994) A receptor for tumor necrosis factor defines an unusual family of cellular and viral proteins. Cell 76:959–962

Stanger BZ, Leder P, Lee T-H, Kim E, Seed B (1995) RIP: a novel protein containing a death domain that interacts with Fas/APO-1 (CD95) in yeast and causes cell death. Cell 81:513–523

Tartaglia LA, Weber RF, Figari IS, Reynolds C, Palladino MA Jr, Goeddel DV (1991) The two different receptors for tumor necrosis factor mediate distinct cellular responses. Proc Natl Acad Sci USA 88:9292–9296

Tartaglia LA, Ayres TM, Wong GHW, Goeddel DV (1993) A novel domain within the 55 kd TNF receptor signals cell death. Cell 74:845–853

Tewari M, Dixit VM (1995) Fas- and Tumor necrosis factor-induced apoptosis is inhibited by the poxvirus crmA gene product. J Biol Chem 270:3255–3260

Tewari M, Quan LT, O'Rourke K, Desnoyers S, Zheng Z, Beidler DR, Poirier GG, Salvesen GS, Dixit VM (1995a) Yama/CPP32β, a mammalian homolog of CED-3, is a crmA-inhibitable protease that cleaves the death substrate poly(ADP-ribose) polymerase. Cell 81:1–20
Tewari M, Beidler DR, Dixit VM (1995b) CrmA-inhibitable cleavage of the 70-kDa protein component of the U1 small nuclear ribonucleoprotein during Fas- and TNF-induced apoptosis. J Biol Chem 270:18738–18741
Watanabe-Fukunaga R, Brannan CI, Copeland NG, Jenkins NA, Nagata S (1992) Lymphoproliferation disorder in mice explained by defects in Fas antigen that mediates apoptosis. Nature 356:314–317
White K, Grether ME, Abrams JM, Young L, Farrell K, Steller H (1994) Genetic control of programmed cell death in Drosophila. Science 264:677–683

Adoptive Immunotherapy in Chimeras

H. J. Kolb

Introduction

Allogeneic bone marrow transplantation is widely used in the treatment of leukaemia and other haematological malignancies. The effectiveness of this method has been demonstrated in patients with advanced and otherwise refractory disease. There are two major modes of action that contribute to the elimination of leukaemia. Transplantation of haematopoietic stem cells provide the possibility of myeloablative regimens as a treatment modality. Total body radiation and some forms of chemotherapy are toxic to stem cells and may thus eliminate leukaemic stem cells independently of their position in the cell cycle. Another important mode of action is an immune reaction directed against neoplastic haematopoietic cells. Allogeneic haematopoietic transplants exhibit a strong graft-versus-leukaemia effect compared with autologous transplants.

The first evidence of a graft-versus-leukaemia effect was provided in mice by Barnes and Loutit (1957). However, the graft-versus-host effect was associated with graft-versus-host disease (GVHD) and mortality due to GVHD in most of the animals. The graft-versus-leukaemia effect was observed in some strain combinations and not in others despite the similar severity of GVHD. Allogeneic bone marrow transplantation was introduced early as a form of adoptive immunotherapy, but its use has been limited by the development of severe GVHD (Mathé et al. 1965a; Mathé et al. 1965b). Evidence of improved survival of patients with chronic GVHD was first provided by the Seattle group (Weiden et al. 1981). Selection of HLA-identical siblings as donors and improved methods for prevention and treatment of GVHD allowed a better survival with less vigorous GVHD. The beneficial effect of GVHD was significant in patients with advanced disease provided that the patients survived 150 days without relapse (Sullivan et al. 1989b). Forty-five percent of patients died early after transplantation and were excluded from the analysis.
The development of GVHD depends on the content of T-cells in the marrow graft. Inactivation and depletion of T cells in the marrow graft effectively prevents GVHD and allows the development of graft-versus-host tolerance in animals and man (Rodt et al. 1984). Unfortunately depletion of T cells increases the risk of leukaemic relapse in patients with chronic myelogenous leukaemia (CML; Apperley et al. 1988; Goldman et al. 1988). The risk of re-

Symposium in Immunology VI
Eibl/Huber/Peter/Wahn (Eds.)

lapse is even increased in patients with acute or chronic GVHD, if the transplant had been depleted of T cells (Horowitz et al. 1990). T-cell depletion does not increase the risk of relapse to the same extent in patients who receive a transplant in an early stage of acute leukaemia (Horowitz et al. 1990).

Several ways have been attempted to improve the anti-leukaemic effect of haematopoietic transplantation. In patients with advanced disease, reducing the intensity of GVHD prophylaxis and infusing donor lymphocytes early after transplantation increased transplant-related toxicity and mortality without reducing the relapse rate (Sullivan et al. 1989a). Similarly, infusion of incremental doses of donor lymphocytes in patients given T-cell-depleted marrow grafts induced acute GVHD without improving leukaemia-free survival significantly (Naparstek et al. 1995). Obviously a therapeutic window is difficult to be defined where a graft-versus-leukaemia reaction occurs without GVHD (Slavin et al. 1992). Induction of chimerism and tolerance followed by adoptive immunotherapy using donor cells appears to be a more promising approach.

Studies in Dogs

Dogs have been widely used in transplantation research. Marrow transplantation studies in dog leukocyte antigen (DLA)-identical littermate dogs have served as a model for the treatment of humans. However leukaemia is rare in dogs and leukaemic dogs are not readily available. We attempted to induce mixed chimerism and to convert mixed chimeras into complete chimeras by adoptive transfer of donor lymphocytes. We asked the following questions: (1) would it be possible to convert mixed into complete chimerism without inducing severe GVHD; (2) can immunity to tetanus toxoid be transferred by transfusion of lymphocytes from sensitized donors; and (3) does transfusion of donor lymphocytes improve the immune reactivity of the canine chimera towards diphtheria toxoid as a new antigen.

Mixed chimerism could be induced in DLA-identical littermate recipients prepared with a single dose of 10 Gy of total body radiation and transfused with a low dose of donor marrow cells (between 1 and 2×10^8 mononuclear cells/kg body weight) treated with absorbed antithymocyte globulin for prevention of GVHD. Dogs not given donor lymphocytes survived without GVHD (Table 1). Dogs transfused with donor lymphocytes (between 2 and 4×10^8) on days 1 and 2 or on days 21 and 22 after transplantation developed severe GVHD and died. Donor lymphocytes transfused more than 60 days after transplantation did not produce GVHD and the dogs survived. Obviously 2 months after transplantation of T-cell-depleted marrow a tolerant state is achieved which cannot be abrogated by transfusion of donor lymphocytes.

Table 1. GVHD and survival after transplantation of antithymocyte-globulin-treated DLA-identical marrow

Donor lymphocyte transfusion – time after marrow transplant	Number of dogs			
	Studied	with GVHD	Alive	Survival time
–	9	0	9	>2 years (all dogs)
Day 1 + 2	2	2	0	51 days, 83 days
Day 21 + 22	2	2	0	56 days, 72 days
Day 61 + 62	7	0	7	>2 years (all dogs)
2 years[a]	1	0	1	>2 years
4.6 years[a]	1	0	1	>2 years

[a] These dogs served as controls for 2 years.

Chimerism was studied by cytogenetic analysis of marrow and phytohaemagglutinin (PHA)-stimulated blood lymphocytes as the donor was of opposite sex to the host. In transfused animals lymphoid chimerism became complete and marrow chimerism converted at a later time (Table 2).

Immunity to tetanus toxoid was transferred by transfusion of donor lymphocytes; transfused dogs showed antibody titres in passive haemagglutination already a week after transfer. After booster injections, high titres persisted for several years in transfused dogs (Fig. 1). In comparison an untransfused dog produced lower titres for a shorter period of time. Vaccination with diphtheria toxoid induced high and persistent titres in transfused animals, whereas the untransfused dog produced only a low titre of antibodies (Fig. 2).

Table 2. Chimerism in marrow and blood

Donor lymphocyte transfusion	% Donor metaphases (Median)			
	<2 months		>2 months	
	marrow	blood	marrow	blood
No	68	38	57	85
Yes	91	21	99	99
Mann-Whitney U test	$p = 0.5$	$p = 0.5$	$p = 0.04$	$p = 0.02$

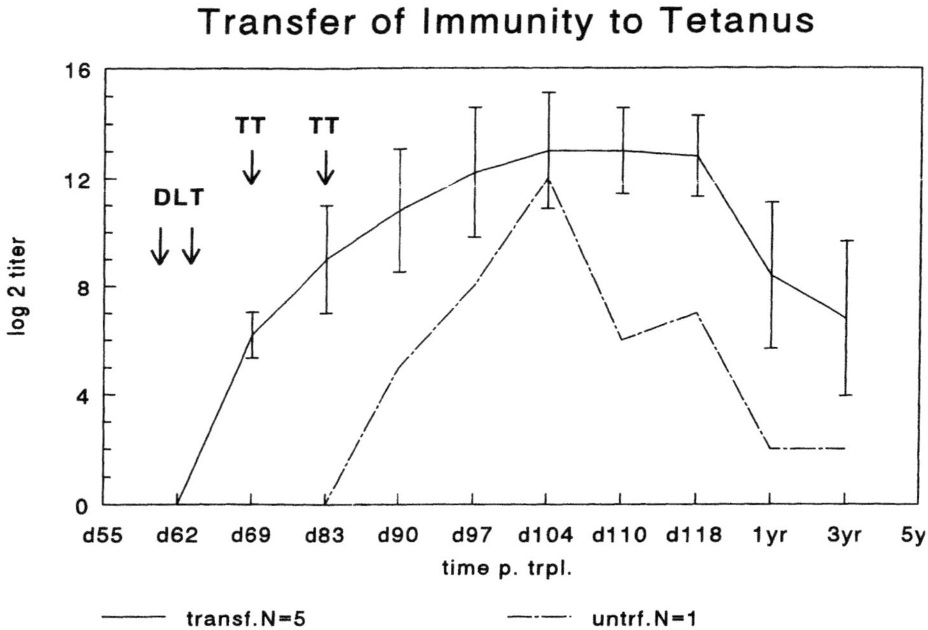

Fig. 1. Immune reactivity to diphtheria toxin (*continuous line*, transfused dogs, $n=5$; *broken line*, untransfused dog, $n=1$)

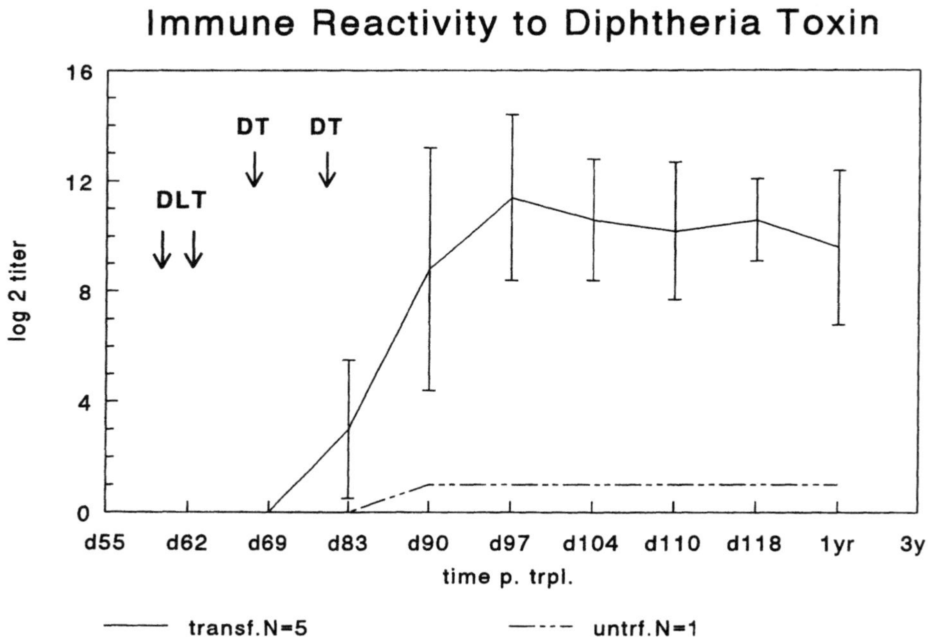

Fig. 2. Immune reactivity to diphtheria toxin (*continuous line*, transfused dogs, $n=5$; *broken line*, untransfused dog, $n=0$)

Treatment of Recurrent Leukaemia by Transfusion of Donor Lymphocytes – Munich Experience

The first patient was treated in October 1988 in Munich (Kolb et al. 1990). This patient had CML in chronic phase and unterwent a transplantation with marrow from his HLA-identical brother in April 1985 and had been a complete chimera. Recurrence of leukaemia was first detected in April 1988 and the disease progressed to haematological relapse in July 1988. He was then treated with interferon-α (INF-α). The blood counts decreased, but his cytogenetic status deteriorated with an increasing proportion of Philadelphia-chromosome-positive cells and a new evolving clone (Table 3). He was given two transfusions of donor leukocyte concentrates and a moderate degree of GVHD occurred 2.5 months after transfusion. GVHD resolved during immunosuppressive treatment. Isoenzyme studies of chimerism showed host type granulocytes and a mixture of donor and host mononuclear cells during relapse. After transfusion of donor lymphocytes, all cells in blood and marrow were of donor type again and Philadelphia-chromosome-positive cells disappeared gradually. Repeated reverse transcriptase polymerase chain reaction (RT-PCR) analyses for bcr/abl transcripts showed a disappearance of malignant cells; the patient has remained leukaemia free since.

Nine patients with recurrent CML were treated with IFN-α and donor lymphocyte transfusions, and complete remission was induced in seven patients (Table 4). A patient in blast crisis failed to respond. The donor of the second patient was a HLA-mismatched sister; severe GVHD occurred early after transplantation and responded to treatment with an immunosuppressive T-cell antibody. GVHD occurred again early after lymphocyte transfusion and required prompt immunosuppressive treatment. A graft-versus-leukaemia effect could not be achieved. Major side effects of donor lymphocyte transfusions were GVHD in four patients and pancytopenia in five patients. Haematopoiesis was restored in two patients following infusion of donor marrow without further conditioning treatment (Fig.3).

Treatment of acute leukaemia and myelodysplastic syndromes was less effective. Three patients with recurrent acute myeloid leukaemia (AML) and five patients with acute lymphocytic leukaemia (ALL) survived more than 30 days and were evaluable for response. Remissions were achieved by induction chemotherapy in three patients with ALL, but leukaemia recurred despite donor lymphocyte transfusions for consolidation. The most convincing graft-versus-leukaemia effect was seen in a patient with AML: only a partial remission was achieved by induction chemotherapy, but a complete remission was induced by donor lymphocyte transfusions. This patient developed moderately severe GVHD and remained in remission for 33 months (data not shown). Subsequently she died of systemic relapse including leukaemic meningiosis.

Table 3. Response of leukaemia and chimerism in patient no. 105

Months after transplant	Clinical condition	Treatment	Chimerism MNC	Blood PMN	RBC	Marrow MNC	Karyotypes (n)	RT-PCR (BCR/ABL)
11	Remission	None	D	D	–	D	Ph1 – (20)	
28	Remission	None	D	D	D	D	Ph1 – (16)	
39	Haematologic relapse	None	M	R	M	–	Ph1 + (2)	
							Ph1 – (14)	
40	Haematologic relapse	INF-α	M	R	M	–	–	
41	Haematologic relapse	INF-α	M	R	M	M	Ph1 + (14)	
43	Haematologic relapse	INF-α +	–	–	R	–	Ph1 + (18)	
		donor lymphocyte transfusion					Ph1 + 14q + (1)	
44	Haematologic relapse	INF-α discontinued	M	R	M	R	Ph1 + 14q + (15)	
44.5	GVHD	–	M	R	–	M	Ph1 + (12)	
							Ph1 – (6)	
45	GVHD	CsA, Pred, Aza	D	M	–	–	Ph1 – (13)	
46.5	GVHD	CsA	D	D	D	–	Ph1 – (16)	negative
48.5	GVHD>	CsA discontinued	D	D	D	D	Ph1 – (12)	
54	Remission	None	–	–	–	–	Ph1 – (10)	
55	Remission	None	–	–	–	–	Ph1 – (10)	
57	Remission	None	D	D	D	–	Ph1 – (10)	
64	Remission	None	D	D	D	–	Ph1p(9)	
67	Remission	None	–	–	–	–	Ph1 – (10)	
72	Remission	None	D	D	D	–	Ph1 – (10)	

82	Remission	None	–	–	–	–	Ph1 – (13)	negative
94	Remission	None	D	D	D	D	Ph1 – (13)	negative
196	Remission	none	–	–	–	–	Ph1 – (20)	negative

MNC, mononuclear cells; PMN, polymorphonuclear neutrophils; RBC, red blood cells; RT-PCR, reverse transcriptase polymerase chain reaction; D, donor; R, recipient; M, mixture of donor and recipient; Ph, Philadelphia chromosome; IFN-α, interferon-α; CsA, cyclosporin A; Pred, prednisone; Aza, azathioprin

Table 4. Results of treatment of recurrent chronic myelogenous leukaemia with transfusion of donor lymphocytes (4/95 Munich)

Patient no.	Relapse	Time after BMT (months)	Chemotherapy	Time after DLT (months)	GVHD>I	Myelosup-pression	Response		
							Haematologic	Cytogenetic	Molecular
105	haematologic	39	No	4	+	–	CR	CR	CR (>78 months)
162	haematologic	24	No	8	–	–	CR	CR	CR (>71 months)
139	haematologic	39	No	4	+	–	CR	CR	CR (>66 months)
268	haematologic	24	No	5	–	+	CR	CR	CR (>29 months)
xxx	haematologic	12	No	8	–	+	CR	n.d.	CR (died 1.7 months)
326	haematologic	13	No	7	+	+	CR	n.d.	CR (died 1.7 months)
284	haematologic	29	No	4	+	+	Aplasia	No	No (died 16 months)
394	acute phase	2	Yes	4	–	(+)	Blast crisis	No	No (died day 16)
342	haematologic	32	No	1	–	+	CR	CR	CR (>20 months)

DLT, donor lymphocyte transfusion; CR, complete remission; n.d., no data.

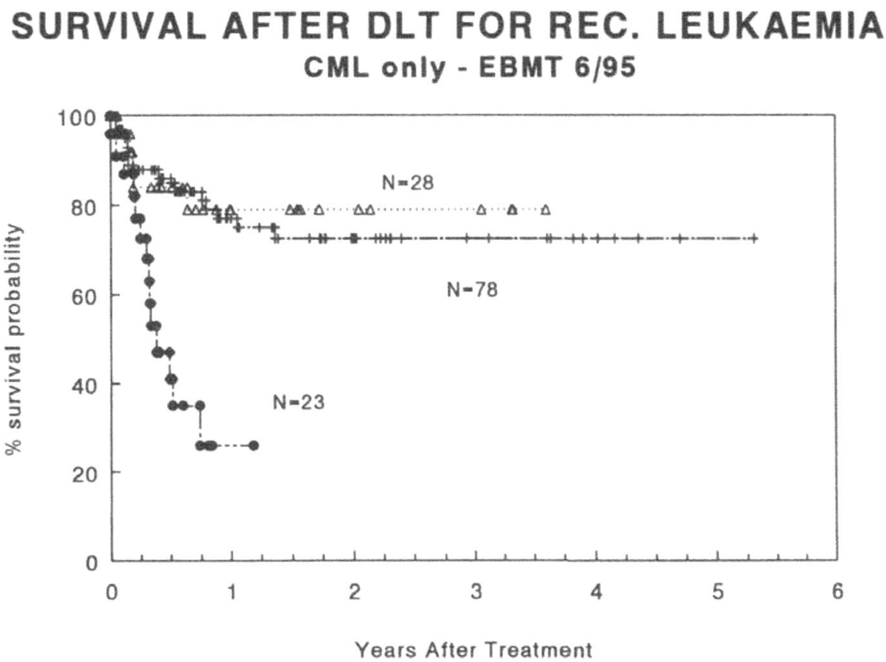

Fig. 3. Survival after donor lymphocyte transfusion for recurrent leukaemia (chronic myeloid leukaemia only; EBMT 6/95). *Triangles*, cytogenetic relapse; *crosses*, haematological relapse; *circles*, transformed relapse

Treatment of Recurrent Leukaemia by Transfusion of Donor Lymphocytes – Experience of the European Group for Blood and Marrow Transplantation

The results of donor lymphocyte transfusions were provided by 49 centres in Europe cooperating in the European Group for Blood and Marrow Transplantation (EBMT). Of the 237 patients reported on, 191 were evaluable for the effect of donor lymphocyte transfusions (Table 5). Best results were obtained in patients with CML in cytogenetic and haematologic relapse. Complete remissions were also achieved in some patients with AML, myelodysplastic syndrome and multiple myeloma. Complete remissions were rare in patients with ALL. Survival prognosis is poor for patients with ALL and best for patients with CML (Fig. 4). There were some ALL patients who responded to donor lymphocyte transfusions not reported by the EBMT study. These patients were exceptional: a young child with an HLA-haploidentical donor (Ferster et al. 1994) and two young children treated as early as 1 month after transplantation (Slavin et al. 1996). In CML, complete cytogenetic responses may be achieved only after several weeks and molecular remissions

Table 5. Graft-versus-leukaemia effect of donor lymphocyte transfusions (EBMT-study 6/95)

Diagnosis	Number of patients: Studied	Evaluable[a]	Complete remission (%)
CML			
Cytogenetic relapse	29	26	19 (73)
Haematologic relapse	79	74	52 (70)
Transformed phase	22	13	1 (8)
Polycythaemia vera	1	1	1
AML	50	39	8 (21)
MDS	9	7	3 (43)
ALL	38	23	1
Multiple myeloma	7	6	1 (16)
NHL	2	2	1
Total number of patients	237	191	86 (45)

CML, chronic myelogenous leukaemia; AML, acute myeloid leukaemia; MDS, myelodysplastic syndrome; ALL, acute lymphocytic leukaemia; NHL, non-Hodgkin's lymphoma.

[a] Patients in remission after chemotherapy and patients surviving less than 30 days after transfusion were exluded from evaluation.

with the absence of *bcr/abl* transcripts as determined by reverse transcription polymerase chain reaction (RT-PCR) may require several months to occur (Van Rhee et al. 1994). Once remissions are attained they appear to be durable. However second relapses do occur and may be treated a second time with success.

The mortality due to the donor lymphocyte transfusion may approach 20%. The main causes of death are GVHD, marrow aplasia or both. Patients should be followed closely for GVHD and marrow aplasia to allow the timely intervention with immunosuppressive therapy and infusion of donor stem cells.

In CML patients the response to donor lymphocyte transfusion correlated with the severity grade of GVHD (Table 6). However GVHD is not a prerequisite for a response of CML, the response rate was 38 % for patients without GVHD and 70 % for patients with mild GVHD not requiring treatment.

Myelosuppression is another side effect that may be related to the response of leukaemia. Myelosuppression was most frequent in patients with haematologic relapse of leukaemia and less frequent in patients with cytogenetic relapse (Table 7). Myelosuppressive effects may not be differentiated from graft-versus-leukaemia effects in patients with most of their haematopoiesis produced by the leukaemic clone. Severe myelosuppression may be

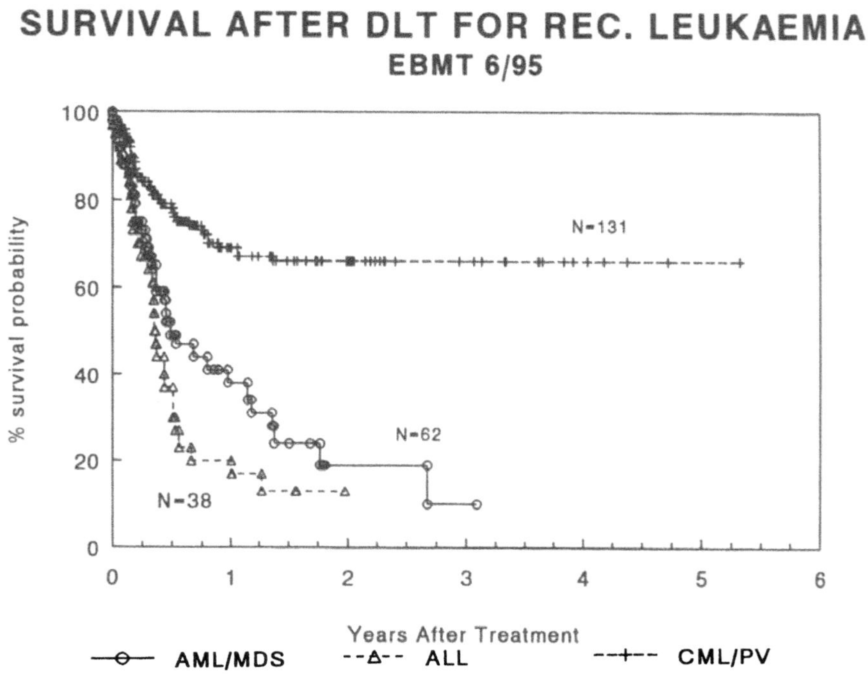

Fig. 4. Survival after donor lymphocyte transfusion for recurrent leukaemia (EBMT 6/95). *Circles*, acute myeloid leukaemia/myelodysplastic syndrome; *triangles*, acute lymphocytic leukaemia; *crosses*, chronic myeloid leukaemia/polycythaemia vera (*PV*)

Table 6. Graft-versus-leukaemia effect[a] of donor lymphocyte transfusions (EBMT-study 6/95)

GVHD-grade	Number of evaluable patients[b]	Number of patients responding (%)
0	39	15 (38%)
I	20	14 (70%)
II	29	27 (93%)
III	12	11 (92%)
IV	7	5 (71%)

[a] Correlation with GVHD in CML-patients (cytogenetic and haematologic relapse).
[b] Patients surviving less than 30 days and in remission after treatment were excluded from the analysis

corrected by the transfusion of marrow from the donor without conditioning (Fig. 5).

The effect of concomitant treatment with IFN-α was studied retrospectively. IFN-α did not improve the response to donor lymphocyte transfusions

Table 7. Myelosuppression after donor lymphocyte transfusions (EBMT-study 6/95). See table 5 for abbreviations

Diagnosis	Number of evaluable patients[a]	Number of patients with pancytopenia (%)
CML		
Cytogenetic relapse	23	4 (17)
Haematologic relapse	72	30 (42)
Transformed phase	3	1 (33)
Polycythaemia vera	1	1
AML	18	10 (56)
MDS	7	2 (29)
ALL	8	2 (25)
Multiple myeloma	4	0

[a] Patients surviving less than 30 days and patients treated with chemotherapy were excluded from the analysis.

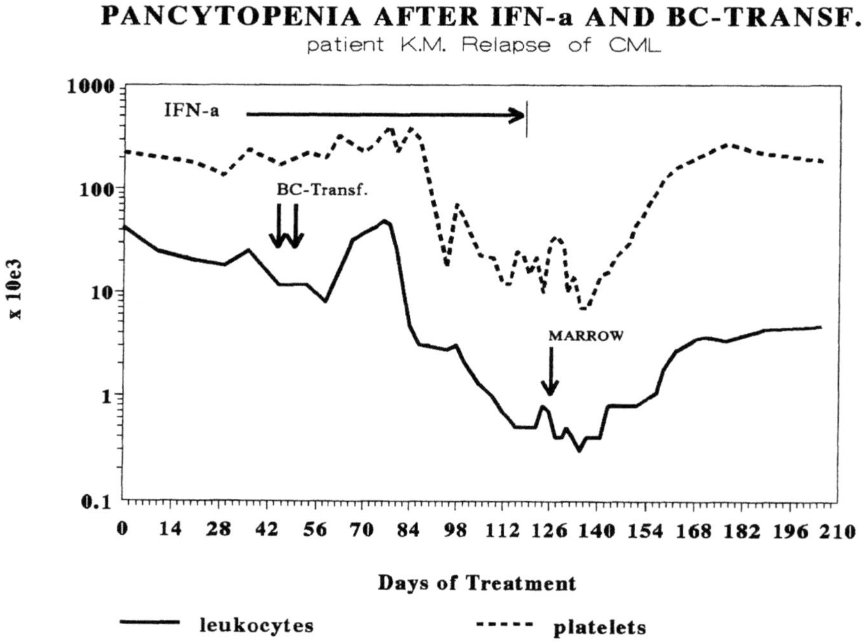

Fig. 5. Pancytopenia after interferon-α and buffy coat (lymphocyte) transfusion. This patient suffered a relapse with chronic myeloid leukaemia (*continuous line*, leukocytes; *dotted line*, platelets)

nor did it increase the severity of GVHD. However patients treated with IFN-α developed cytopenia more frequently than patients given donor lymphocytes without IFN-α (Table 8). However, evaluation of the effects of IFN-α may have been biased by the selection of patients for donor lymphocyte transfusion after IFN-α treatment had failed. Some patients treated by the Sloane Kettering Group responded to donor lymphocytes only after concomitant treatment with IFN-α (Mackinnon et al. 1995).

Preventing Graft-Versus-Host Disease Following Donor Lymphocyte Transfusions

In contrast to the results in animals GVHD develops in humans after donor lymphocyte transfusions. Forty-one percent of all patients and 61% of responding patients develop GVHD of grade II and higher. Prophylactic immunosuppressive treatment prevented GVHD after lymphocyte transfusion, but it ablated the graft-versus-leukaemia effect at the same time (Jiang et al. 1993). Other investigators transfused incremental doses of T cells starting at very low levels (Mackinnon et al. 1995) or depleted CD8-positive T cells from the inoculum (Giralt et al. 1995). Both approaches had some success; 1×10^7 T cells was the lowest effective dose where only one of eight patients developed GVHD. Following transfusion of CD8-depleted T cells, GVHD was observed in only three of ten patients. These approaches should be evaluated in a larger number of patients.

Table 8. Effect of interferon-α on donor lymphocyte transfusions in chronic myelogenous leukaemia patients (EBMT 6/95)

	Interferon treatment		
	Yes (*n*)	No (*n*)	*p*-value[a]
Complete remission			
Yes (%)	49 (75)	16	
No (%)	20 (71)	8	N.S.
GVHD>grade I			
Yes (%)	33 (50)	33	
No (%)	13 (43)	17	N.S.
Myelosuppression			
Yes (%)	27 (42)	38	
No (%)	7 (24)	22	$p=0.08$

[a] Fisher exact test

Improving the Response of Acute Leukaemia and Chronic Myelogenous Leukaemia in Transformation

There are several variables that possibly influence the response to adoptive immunotherapy with donor lymphocytes. Most important is the time required for the graft-versus-leukaemia reaction to eliminate residual leukaemic cells. In chronic phase CML, there is sufficient time for the reaction to build up and eliminate residual CML cells. In acute leukaemia, progression of leukaemic growth may be so fast that the graft-versus-leukaemia reaction may not overcome leukaemic growth. In multiple myeloma, growth of neoplastic cells is also slow enough to allow a graft-versus-leukaemia reaction to attain control (Verdonck et al. 1996).

Another variable is the maturation stage attained by the neoplastic cells and their potential to present antigen in an immunogenic way. In the chronic phase of CML, leukaemic cells differentiate to mature cells including dendritic cells carrying the malignant phenotype. In some cases AML cells may differentiate to mature cells including dendritic cells, the most potent antigen-presenting cells. Differentiation may be facilitated by a prior reduction of the tumour mass (Mittermüller et al. 1986).

Dendritic cells may be produced in vitro by culturing CD34 positive progenitor cells (Romani et al. 1994; Caux et al. 1992) in the presence of granulocyte-macrophage-colony stimulating factor (GM-CSF), tumour necrosis factor-α (TNF-α) and interleukin-4 (IL-4). Bone-marrow-derived antigen-presenting cells can present tumour antigens in a MHC-class-I-restricted manner (Huang et al. 1994). Therefore, transfusion of dendritic cells or haematopoietic progenitor cells and treatment with GM-CSF may compensate for insufficient presentation of antigen by the leukaemic cells. We have treated five patients with mobilised blood stem cells and lymphocytes and GM-CSF. Two patients with ALL received intensive chemotherapy suitable for conditioning and one remained in remission for more than one year. Three patients with AML were treated with less intensive chemotherapy and received blood stem cells followed by treatment with GM-CSF. Two patients responded and one patient had a transient reduction of myelosarcoma. One patient is now 10 months after treatment with donor blood stem cells and GM-CSF during a partial remission which was induced with low dose cytosine arabinoside (Fig. 6). In a patient with ALL, leukaemia progressed in the presence of vigorous GVHD. In this patient escape mechanisms of leukaemic cells must be considered.

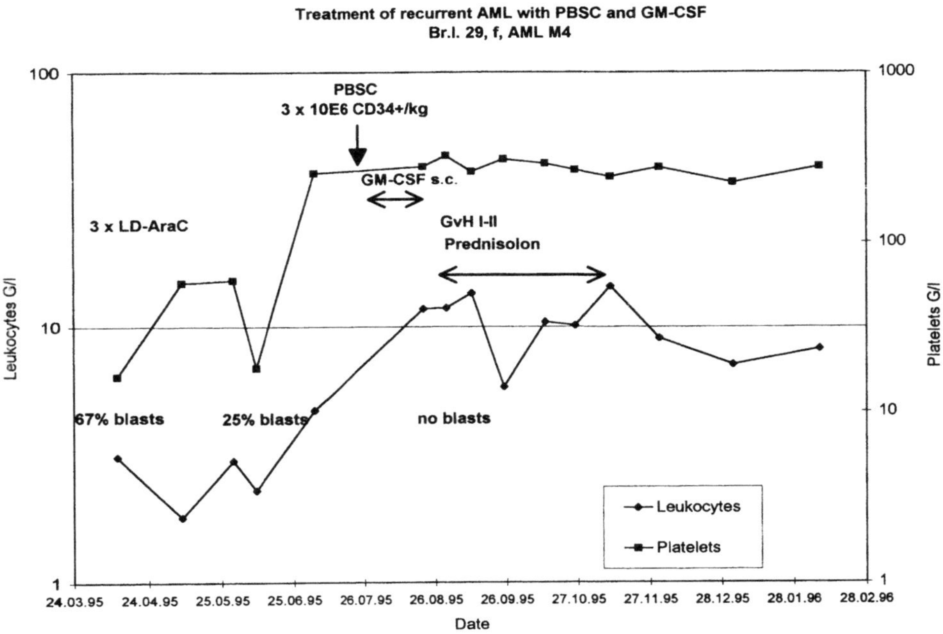

Fig. 6. Treatment of recurrent acute myeloid leukaemia with peripheral blood stem cells (*PBSC*) and granulocyte/macrophage-colony stimulating factor (*GM-CSF*).

Possible Mechanisms of Graft-Versus-Leukaemia Reactions and of Immune Escape

Donor lymphocytes are transfused into a tolerant and chimeric host. The success of the adoptive immunotherapy depends on the tolerant state of the host. Patients without evidence of persistent chimerism do not respond as well as chimeric patients to donor lymphocyte transfusions (Schattenberg et al. 1996). Unlike experimental animals, humans may develop GVHD after donor lymphocyte transfusions even if they are in a chimeric and tolerant state. Experimental animals are young and in their early adulthood when they are used. Most patients are in a later stage of their life at the time of transplantation. Frequently, patients and their donors may be sensitized by pregnancies and have been exposed to a great number of viruses that may initiate immune reactions. Finally, the leukaemia may produce proinflammatory cytokines and stimulate transfused donor cells.

Donor lymphocytes may recognize histocompatibility antigens and leukaemia-specific antigens in the host. The BCR–ABL fusion peptide is specific for leukaemia cells in CML and Philadelphia-positive ALL. Several groups of investigators have shown proliferative and cytotoxic T-cell responses after immunisation in vitro (Chen et al. 1992; Mannering et al. 1996). However evidence for leukaemia-specific reactions in vivo has not been provided yet. Present evidence supports a reaction against histocompatibility antigens, since lymphocytes from syngeneic twins were not effective against recurrent CML (Bunjes et al. 1996). Reactions against minor histocompatibility antigens may not necessarily be associated with GVHD since some minor histocompatibility antigens are predominantly expressed on haematopoietic cells (Goulmy et al. 1993). The graft-versus-host reaction against haematopoietic cells may be sufficiently specific as haematopoietic stem cells are provided by the graft. Another mechanism may also provide leukaemia specificity by the different proliferative state of leukaemic cells compared with normal stem cells (Kolb et al. 1996). In patients with CML under treatment, leukaemic cells are predominantly DR-positive and normal stem cells are enriched in the DR-negative fraction (Verfaillie et al. 1992). DR-restricted T cells recognize leukaemic cells and spare DR-negative normal stem cells. Adhesion molecules on leukaemic cells may guide the reaction via specific ligands, and cytokines produced by leukaemic cells may sustain the graft-versus-leukaemia reaction (Duncombe et al. 1989).

However there are also several possibilities as to why leukaemic cells can escape strong immune reactions like graft-versus-host reactions. Expression of HLA class I and class II antigens may be decreased, and leukaemic cells may not be recognized by donor T cells. Indeed the level of antigen expression is frequently lower, but the expression of single allelic antigens may be of greater importance, since specific peptides bind with varying avidity. Insufficient expression of adhesion molecules and costimulatory signals impair reactivity and induce tolerance. Cytokines play an important role in the regulation of the reaction. Insufficient production of proinflammatory cytokines allows leukaemia cells to escape immune control and leads to inadequate production of inhibitory cytokines.

Perspectives of Adoptive Immunotherapy in Chimeras

In recent years much experience has been gained in the use of donor lymphocytes for adoptive immunotherapy of recurrent leukaemia. GVHD is controlled in most HLA-identical donor recipient combinations at least as effectively as in marrow transplantation. Unfortunately chimerism is a precondition for successful adoptive immunotherapy. However, adoptive immunotherapy at a later time provides the possibility to treat leukaemia in a two-step fashion. The first step is inducing transplantation tolerance, and the second step involves immunotherapy. Future conditioning regimens will allow for a minimum of chemotherapy and radiotherapy necessary for engraftment and disregard elimination of all tumour cells at once. As toxic conditioning regimens are not necessary for immunotherapy the treatment may be repeated several times.

Selectivity against leukaemia cells may be achieved by immunization of donor lymphocytes in vitro against leukaemia-specific antigens or minor histocompatibility antigens present on haematopoietic cells. Transfer of suicide genes into T cells has been advocated for the interruption of graft-versus-host reactions and a better control of immunotherapy (Tiberghien et al. 1994).

Adoptive immunotherapy has been used for the treatment of viral infections and EBV-induced tumours (Papadopoulos et al. 1994; Rooney et al. 1994). T cells of immune and genetically non-susceptible donors could be used for the treatment of persistent viral infections and autoimmune diseases.

Acknowledgements. The author expresses his gratitude to the following transplant centres for providing their results for evaluation: Barcelona, Basel, Berlin, Besançon, Bologna, Bolzano, Brussels (J. Bordet), Brussels (St. Luc), Copenhagen, Creteil (H. Mondor), Dublin (St. James), Düsseldorf, Freiburg, Geneva, Graz, Hamburg, Hanover, Helsinki Haematology, Homburg/Saar, Huddinge, Innsbruck, Idar-Oberstein, Jerusalem, Kiel, Leicester Royal Inf., Leiden Haematology, London Charing Cross, London Hammersmith, London Royal Free, Leipzig, Madrid, Mainz, Manchester Ped., Munich, Nancy, Napoli, Nijmegen, Oslo, Pavia, Riyadh, Rome (La Sapienza), Rome (San Cuore); Rotterdam DDHK, Santander, Tübingen, Ulm, Utrecht, Zagreb, Zürich.

References

Antin JH (1993) Graft-versus-leukemia: no longer an epiphenomenon. Blood 82:2273–2277

Apperley JF, Mauro FR, Goldman JM et al. (1988) Bone marrow transplantation for chronic myeloid leukemia in first chronic phase: importance of a graft-versus-leukemia effect. Br J Haematol 69:239–245

Barnes DHW, Loutit JF (1957) Treatment of murine leukaemia with X-rays and homologous bone marrow. Br J Haematol 3:241–252

Caux C, Dezutter-Dambuyant C, Schmitt D, Banchereau J (1992) GM-CSF and TNF-α cooperate in the generation of dendritic Langerhans cells. Nature 360:258–261

Chen W, Peace BJ, Rovira DK, You SG, Cheever MA (1992) T-cell immunity to the joining region of p210 BCR-ABL protein. Proc Natl Acad Sci USA 89:1468–1471

Drobyski WR, Roth MS, Thibodeau SN, Gottschall JL (1992) Molecular remission occurring after donor leukocyte infusions for the treatment of relapsed chronic myelogenous leukemia after allogeneic bone marrow transplantation. Bone Marrow Transplant 10:301–304

Drobyski WR, Keever CA, Roth MS, Koethe S, Hanson G, McFadden P, Gottschall JR,Ash RC, van Tuinen P, Horowitz MM, Flomenberg N (1993) Salvage immunotherapy using donor leukocyte infusions as treatment for relpased chronic myelogenous leukemia after bone marrow transplantation: Efficacy and toxicity of a defined T-cell dose. Blood 82:2310–2318

Duncombe AS, Heslop HE, Turner M, Meager A, Priest R, Exley T, Brenner MK (1989) Tumor necrosis factor mediates autocrine growth inhibition in a chronic leukemia. J Immunol 143:3828–3834

Ferster A, Bujan W, Mouraux T, Devalck C, Heimann P, Sariban E (1994) Complete remission following donor leukocyte infusion in ALL relapsing after haploidentical bone marrow transplantation. Bone Marrow Transplant 14:331-332

Frassoni F, Fagioli F, Sessarego M, Gualandi F, van Lint MT, Lamparelli T, Occhini D,

Figari O, Valbonesi M, Bacigalupo A (1992) The effect of donor leukocyte infusion in patients with leukemia following allogeneic bone marrow transplantation. Exp Hematol 20:712 (abstract)

Giralt S, Hester J, Huh Y, Hirsch-Ginsberg C, Rondon G, Seong D, Lee M, Gajewski J, Van Besien K, Khouri I, Mehra R, Przepiorka D, Körbling M, Talpaz M, Kantarjian H, Fischer H, Deisseroth A, Champlin R (1995) CD8-depleted donor lymphocyte infusion as treatment for relapsed chronic myelogenous leukemia after allogeneic bone marrow transplantation. Blood 86:4337–4343

Goldman JM, Galt RP, Horowitz MM, Biggs JC, Champlin RE, Gluckman E, Hoffmann RG, Jacobsen SJ, Marmont AM, McGlave PB, Messner HA, Rimm AA, Rozman C, Speck B, Tura S, Weiner RS, Bortin MM (1988) Bone marrow transplantation for chronic myelogenous leukemia in chronic phase: Increased risk of relapse associated with T-cell depletion. Ann Intern Med 108:806

Goulmy E (1993) Minor H antigens: a „1993" look into their perspectives. Bone Marrow Transplant 12 (Suppl 4):9–10

Hertenstein B, Wiesneth M, Novotny J, Bunjes D, Stefanic M, Heinze B, Hübner G, Heimpel H, Arnold R (1993) Interferon alpha and donor buffy coat transfusions for treatment of relapsed chronic myeloid leukemia after allogeneic marrow transplantation. Transplantation 56:1114–1118 (abstract)

Horowitz MM, Gale RP, Sondel PM, Goldman JM, Kersey J, Kolb HJ, Rimm AA, Ringden O, Rozman C, Speck B et al (1990) Graft-versus-leukemia reactions after bone marrow transplantation. Blood 75:555–562

Huang AYC, Golumbek P, Ahmadzadeh M, Jaffee E, Pardoll D, Levitsky H (1994) Role of bone marrow-derived cells presenting MHC class I-restricted tumor antigens. Science 264:961–965

Jiang YZ, Cullis JO, Kanfer, EJ, Goldman JM, Barrett AJ (1993) T cell and NK cell mediated graft-versus-leukaemia reactivity following donor buffy coat transfusion to treat relapse after marrow transplantation for chronic myeloid leukaemia. Bone Marrow Transplant 11:133–138

Kolb HJ, Mittermueller J, Clemm C, Ledderose G, Brehm G, Heim M, Wilmanns W (1990) Donor leukocyte transfusions for treatment of recurrent chronic myelogenous leukemia in marrow transplant patients. Blood 76:2462-2465

Kolb HJ, Beisser K, Mittermueller J et al (1992) Adoptive immunotherapy in human and canine chimeras. In: Hiddemann W, Büchner T, Plunkett W et al. (eds.) Acute Leukemias – Pharmakokinetics. Springer, Berlin Heidelberg New York pp 595–600

Kolb HJ, Schattenberg A, Goldman JM, Hertenstein B, Jacobsen N, Arcese W, Ljungman P, Ferrant A, Verdonck L, Niederwieser D, van Rhee F, Mittermüller J, De Witte T, Holler E, Ansari H (1995) Graft-versus-leukemia effect of donor lymphocyte transfusions in marrow grafted patients. Blood 86:2041–2050

Kolb HJ, Mittermüller J, Holler E, Thalmeier K, Bartram CR (1996) Graft-versus-host reaction spares normal stem cells in chronic myelogenous leukemia. Bone Marrow Transplant 17:449–452

Mackinnon S, Papadopoulos EB, Carabasi MH, Reich L, Collins NH, Boulad F, Castro-Malaspina H, Childs BH, Gillio AP, Kernan NA, Small TM, Young JW, OReilly RJ (1995) Adoptive immunotherapy evaluating escalating doses of donor leukocytes for relapse of chronic myeloid leukemia after bone marrow transplantation: separation of graft-versus-leukemia responses from graft-versus-host disease. Blood 86:1261–1268

Mannering SI, McKenzie JL, Hart DN (1996) Generation of T-lymphocyte clones specific for the BCR-ABL fusion peptide presented by dendritic cells and other antigen presenting cells. Bone Marrow Transplant 17 (Suppl 1): S59 (abstract)

Mathé G, Amiel JL, Schwartzenberg L, Cattan A, Schneider M, De Vries JM, Tubiana M, Lalanne C, Binet JL, Papiernik M, Seman G, Matsukuba M, Mery AM, Schwarzmann V, Flaisler A (1965a) Successful allogeneic bone marrow transplantation in man: Chimerism, induced specific tolerance and possible antileukemic effects. Blood 25:179

Mathé G, Amiel JL, Schwarzenberg L, Cattan A, Schneider M (1965b) Adoptive immunotherapy of acute leukemia: Experimental and clinical results. Cancer Res 25:1525–1530

Mittermüller J, Kolb HJ, Gerhartz HH, Wilmanns W (1986) In vivo differentiation of leukemic blasts and effect of low dose ara-c in a marrow grafted patient with leukemic relapse. Br J Haematol 62:757–762

Naparstek E, Or R, Nagler A, Cividalli G, Engelhard D, Aker M, Gimon Z, Manny N, Sacks T, Tochner Z, Weiss L, Samual S, Brautbar C, Hale G, Waldmann H, Steinberg SM (1995) T-cell depleted allogeneic bone marrow transplantation for acute leukaemia using Campath-1 antibodies and post-transplant administration of donors' peripheral blood lymphocytes for prevention of relapse. Br J Haematol 89:506–515

Papadopoulos EB, Ladanyi M, Emanuel D, Mackinnon S, Boulad F, Carabasi MH, Castro-Malaspina H, Childs BH, Gillio AP, Small TN, Young JW, Kernan NA, OReilly RJ (1994) Infusions of donor leukocytes to treat Epstein-Barr virus-associated lymphoproliferative disorders after allogeneic bone marrow transplantation. N Engl J Med 330:1185–1191

Porter DL, Roth MS, McGarigle C, Ferrara JLM, Antin JH (1994) Induction of graft-versus-host disease as immunotherapy for relapsed chronic myeloid leukemia. New Engl J Med 330:100–106

Romani N, Gruner S, Brang D, Kämpgen E, Lenz A, Trockenbacher B, Konwalinka G, Fritsch PO, Steinman RM, Schuler G (1994) Proliferating dendritic cell progenitors in human blood. J Exp Med 180:83–93

Rooney CM, Loftin SK, Brenner MK, Heslop HE (1994) Early detection and treatment of EBV-associated post transplant lymphoproliferative disease. EBMT Congress, Harrogate, UK, March 13–16, 1994, BMT:136 (abstract 167)

Rodt, H, Kolb HJ, Netzel B, Hoffman-Fezer, G Thierfelder S (1984) Serological prevention of graft-versus-host disease: an experimental and clinical survey. In: Slavin S (ed) Tolerance in bone marrow and organ transplantation, pp 253–285

Schattenberg A, van de Wiel-van Kemenade E, Schaap N, De Witte T (1996) Chimerism and outcome of the infusion of lymphocytes as a treatment for relapse after T cell depleted BMT. Bone Marrow Transplant 17 (Suppl 1): S9 (abstract)

Slavin S, Ackerstein A, Weiss L, Nagler A, Or R, Naparstek E (1992) Immunotherapy of minimal residual disease by immunocompetent lymphocytes and their activation by cytokines. Cancer Invest 10:221-227

Slavin S, Naparstek E, Nagler A, Ackerstein A, Samuel S, Kapelushnik J, Brautbar C, Or R (1996) Allogeneic cell therapy with donor peripheral blood cells and recombinant human interleukin-2 to treat leukemia relapse after allogeneic bone marrow transplantation. Blood 87:2195–2204

Sullivan KM, Storb R, Buckner CD, Fefer A, Fisher L, Weiden PL, Witherspoon RP, Appelbaum FR, Babaji M, Hansen J, Martin P, Sanders JE, Singer J, Thomas ED (1989a) Graft-versus-host disease as adoptive immunotherapy in patients with advanced hematologic neoplasms. N Engl J Med 320:828–834

Sullivan KM, Weiden PL, Storb R, Witherspoon RP, Fefer A, Fisher L, Buckner CD, Anasetti C, Appelbaum FR, Badger C, Beatty P, Bensinger W, Berenson R, Bigelow C, Cheever MA, Clift RA, Deeg HJ, Doney K, Greenberg P, Hansen JA, Hill R, Loughran T, Martin P, Neiman PE, Petersen FB, Sanders J, Singer J, Stewart P, Thomas ED (1989b) Influence of acute and chronic graft-versus-host disease on relapse and survival after bone marrow transplantation from HLA-identical siblings as treatment of acute and chronic leukemia. Blood 73:1720–1728

Szer J, Grigg AP, Phillips GL, Sheridan WP (1993) Donor leukocyte infusions after chemotherapy for patients relapsing with acute leukaemia following allogeneic BMT. Bone Marrow Transplant 11:109–111

Tiberghien P, Reynolds CW, Keller J, Spence S, Deschaseaux M, Certou JM, Contassot E, Murphy WJ, Lyons R, Chiang Y et al (1994) Ganciclovir treatment of herpes simplex thymidine kinase-transduced primary T lymphocytes: an approach for specific in vivo T-cell depletion after bone marrow transplantation. Blood 84:1333–1341

van Rhee F, Lin F, Cullis JO, Spencer A, Cross NCP, Chase A, Garicochea B, Bungey J, Barrett AJ, Goldman JM (1994) Relapse of chronic myeloid leukemia after allogeneic bone marrow transplant: The case for giving donor leukocyte transfusions before the onset of hematological relapse. Blood 83:3377–3383

Verdonck LF, Lokhorst HM, Dekker AW, Nieuwenhuis HK, Petersen EF (1996) Graft-versus-myeloma effect in two cases. Lancet 347:800–801

Verfaillie CM, Miller WJ, Boylan K, McGlave PB (1992) Selection of benign primitive hematopoietic progenitors in chronic myelogenous leukemia on the basis of HLA-DR antigen expression. Blood 79:1003–1010

Weiden PL, Storb R, Tsoi M-S, Graham TC, Lerner KG, Thomas ED (1976) Infusion of donor lymphocytes into stable canine radiation chimeras: Implications for mechanism of transplantation tolerance. J Immunol 116:1212–1219

Weiden PL, Sullivan KM, Flournoy N, Storb R, Thomas ED, The Seattle Marrow Transplant Team (1981) Antileukemic effect of chronic graft-versus-host disease. Contribution to improved survival after allogeneic marrow transplantation. N Engl J Med 304:1529–1531

Towards the Development of Immunogenic Colon Cancer Cells for Immunotherapy

S. Meuer, W. Rudy, A. Habicht, M. Lindauer, and U. Moebius

Introduction

Colorectal cancer as opposed to melanoma or renal cancer is considered a nonimmunogenic type of malignancy. Nonimmunogenicity of tumor cells is believed to be the result of either a failure to induce resting pre-effector T lymphocytes to differentiate into effector cells or active mechanisms of immunosuppression which are exerted by tumor cells as soluble inhibitory activities. One must expect that both mechanisms play a role in the interaction between malignant tissue and the host immune system.

Recently, several components required for an induction of specific cellular immune responses were identified. These are specific ligands of receptor structures through which lymphocytes receive signals for their activation and differentiation [1–6]. In addition to antigen recognition (peptide/HLA complex) by the T-cell antigen receptor, additional signals that can be mediated through a series of accessory receptors including CD2, CD4, CD8, and CD28 have to be present for lymphocyte activation (Fig. 1). Antigen recognition in the absence of accessory receptor costimulation leads to a stage of T-cell anergy or even to T-cell deletion by apoptosis [7–11]. Thus, one reason for nonimmunogenicity of tumor cells could be their lack of expression of appropriate copy numbers of ligands for accessory receptors and as a consequence failure to costimulate tumor-recognizing T cells [12, 13].

We have tested this hypothesis, employing two cell lines derived from human colon cancer. These cell lines were selected because they do not secrete molecules which inhibit T-cell proliferation and because they express the frequent allele HLA A2.1. Our goal was to create immunogenic colon cancer cells by somatic gene transfer. This would, for the first time, provide tools for

1. identifying unknown tumor antigens of colon cancer;
2. tumor cell vaccination, i.e., attempts to induce immune responses in vivo.

Symposium in Immunology VI
Eibl/Huber/Peter/Wahn (Eds.)

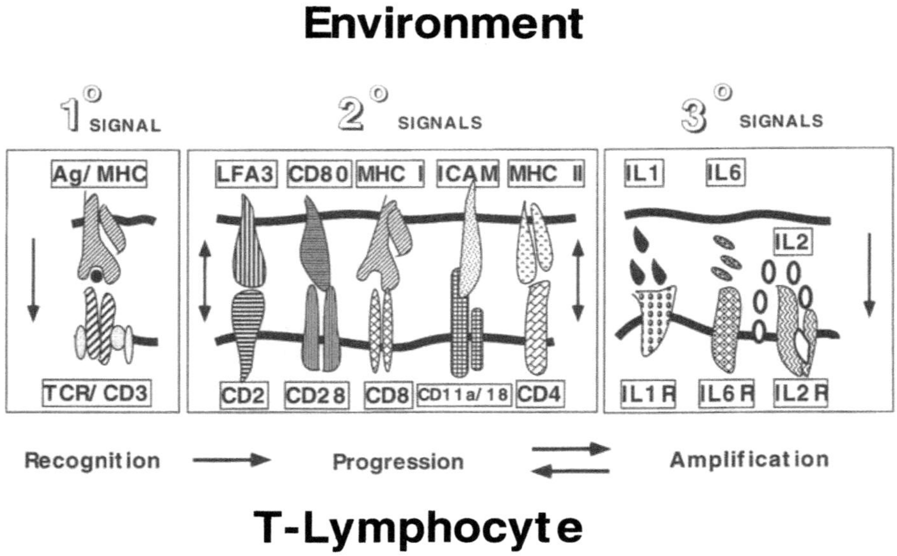

Fig. 1. Hierarchy of signals involved in T-lymphocyte activation. Schematic representation of receptors and ligands. This graphic depicts the T-cell plasma membrane (*bottom*) and the plasma membrane of an antigen-presenting cell (*top*)

Wild Type Tumor Cell Lines do not Activate Resting Human T Lymphocytes in the Allogeneic Mixed Lymphocyte Tumor Cell Culture

Established epithelial tumor cell lines from colorectal carcinoma (SW480, SW707) and melanoma (Mz19, SkMel63) were tested for their capacity to activate T lymphocytes in vitro. To this end peripheral blood T lymphocytes from healthy donors were incubated with the various cell lines and subsequently DNA synthesis by responding T lymphocytes was determined by means of ^{3}H-labeled thymidine incorporation. As a control, the known immunogenic Epstein-Barr virus (EBV)-transformed B lymphoplastoid cell line (BLCL), M7, was employed. Normally, in such a situation T lymphocytes on recognizing alloantigens should respond with proliferation. However, T cells from different healthy donors are not activated in vitro under these conditions (except in the case of the BLCL-M7). Note that coculture of epithelial tumor cells with BLCL-M7 cells in an allogeneic mixed lymphocyte tumor cell culture (MLTC) did not suppress the M7-directed T-cell response indicating that these tumor cells did not actively suppress T-cell proliferation (not shown).

Table 1. Immunofluorescence analysis of tumor cell lines

Cell line	Negative control	Class-I-MHC	Class-II-MHC	CD54	CD58	CD80	CD86
SW480	3.1[a]	74.3	3.0	3.2	19.8	3.0	3.2
SW707	2.8	98.3	3.2	3.3	14.8	2.8	2.8
MzMel9	2.8	27.2	2.9	8.0	5.6	2.9	2.7
SkMel63	2.0	33.6	18.8	12.8	4.2	1.9	2.1
M7	2.7	353.3	86.8	7.5	17.5	20.5	23.1

[a] Mean fluorescence intensity, linear unit. Neg, negative control

The phenotypic characterization of tumor cell lines demonstrated that significant levels of class I MHC molecules are present on their cell surface. This is particularly true for the two colorectal cell lines SW480 and SW707. In addition, these cell lines express reasonable levels of the adhesion molecule CD58, the ligand for the T-cell coreceptor CD2. In contrast, however, expression of CD54 (ligand of CD11a/18) and class II MHC was rather low. Moreover, neither CD80 nor CD86 were detectable by flow cytometric analysis (Table 1).

Expression of CD80 Alone is not Sufficient to Reconstitute Immunogenicity

CD80 is a cell surface antigen which serves as a ligand for the T cell coreceptor CD28 [3–5]. The interaction between CD80 and CD28 is known to provide strong costimulatory signals for primary T-cell activation. To investigate whether expression of CD80 on tumor cells would reconstitute immunogenicity we transfected a CD80 cDNA into two colorectal carcinoma cell lines (SW480, SW707) and one melanoma cell line (SkMel63).

Figure 2 demonstrates that CD80 cell surface levels of at least one clone derived from each of the tumor cell lines was comparable to that typically found on constitutively CD80-positive B-LCL-M7. Subsequently, the various CD80-transfected tumor cells were tested for their ability to induce DNA synthesis of allogeneic T lymphocytes freshly prepared from the blood of healthy donors. As shown in Fig. 3, CD80 transfection into melanoma cells promoted T-cell proliferation up to six-fold compared with the untransfected wild-type cell [14]. This occurs already at low levels of CD80 expression indicating that there is a minimum amount of CD80 expression required for the induction of functional effects. In marked contrast to melanoma transfectants, expression of CD80 in both colon cancer cell lines had no effect on T-cell activation. All CD80 transfectants of SW480 and SW707 were capable of promoting T-cell proliferation in concert with submitogenic concentra-

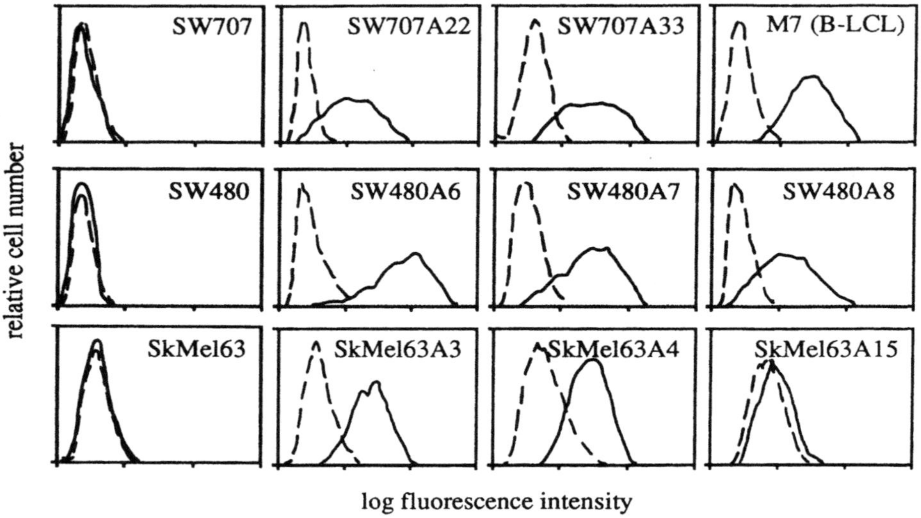

Fig. 2. Immunofluorescence analysis of individual CD80-transfected tumor cell sublines in comparison with the BLCL-M7. Cells were incubated either with a negative control ascites (*dashed line*) or the CD80-specific monoclonal antibody (mAb) 104, followed by incubation with a FITC-labeled secondary mAb

tions of the CD3 monoclonal antibody (OKT3) or phorbol myristate acetate demonstrating that the CD80 molecules expressed on these cells through gene transfer were functionally active. T-cell proliferation induced by CD80 transfected melanoma cells was inhibited by a CD80-specific monoclonal antibody which confirms that growth promotion observed with these cells was related to their expression of CD80.

Coexpression of CD80 and MHC II Does Not Lead to T-Cell Activation

One prominent phenotypic difference between melanoma cells and colorectal carcinoma cell lines is that SkMel63 cells express class II MHC gene products, whereas SW480 and SW707 do not (Table l). To eliminate the possibility that the lack of class II MHC expression is responsible for the failure of colon cancer cells to stimulate T cells in vitro (despite CD80 expression), we transfected cDNA encoding DRα and DRβ3 into SW480 and the CD80 transfectant of SW480 (SW480A6). Analysis by means of flow cytometry demonstrated two clones expressing HLA-DR3 and two additional SW480 subclones coexpressing CD80 and HLA-DR3. The level of HLA-DR3 expression on transfected cells was approximately three to four times lower than the level

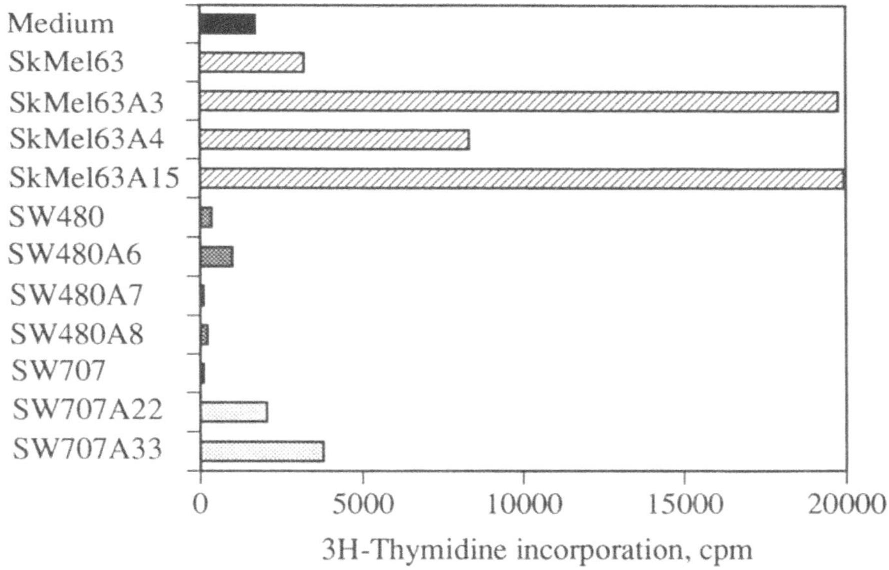

Fig. 3. T-lymphocyte proliferation following stimulation with CD80-transfected melanoma cells. 10^5 resting peripheral blood lymphocytes were incubated with 10^4 irradiated tumor cells (*SkMel63:* melanoma; *SW480, SW707:* colorectal cancer) in 1 ml culture medium for 5 days. Subsequently, T-cell proliferation was determined by ^{3}H-labeled thymidine incorporation. CD80-transfected sublines are indicated with "A"

of class II MHC molecules found on the lymphoblastoid B cell line M7 but was comparable to class II expression on melanoma cells (Fig. 4).

When HLA-DR3-transfected SW480 cells and the subclones coexpressing HLA-DR3 plus CD80 molecules were investigated for their capacity to produce primary T-cell activation in allogeneic MLTC experiments, again no functional effect was observed (not shown).

CD80 and CD86

Recently, a second ligand of CD28, namely CD86, was identified and is proposed to provide costimulation through interaction with its receptor on T lymphocytes [15–17]. As yet it is unclear whether the functional activities of CD80 and CD86 are identical, similar, or completely different. To try to address this point, we generated stable transfectants with a plasmid containing CD86 cDNA. In addition, we transfected CD86 cDNA into SW480 cells which were previously transfected with CD80 (SW480A6). As judged from an immunofluorescence analysis of various subclones (Fig. 5) that were deri-

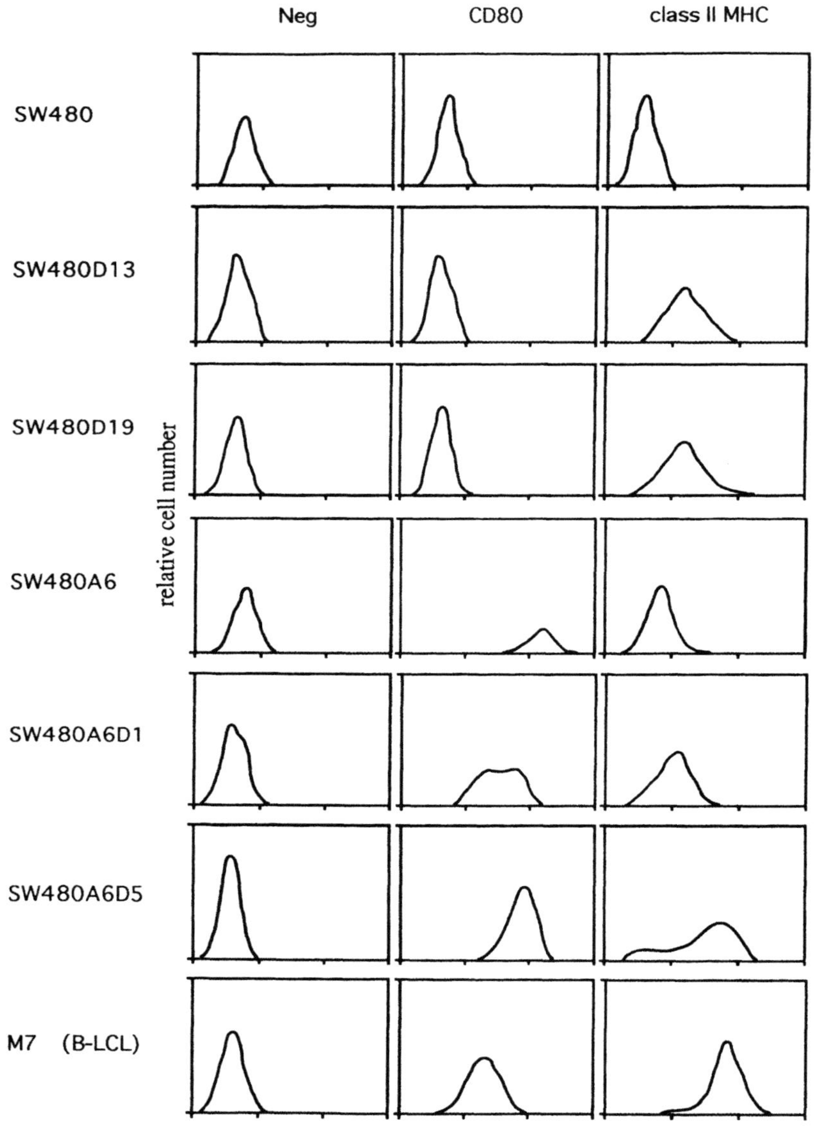

Fig. 4. Immunofluorescence analysis of HLA-DR3-transfected variants of SW480 and SW480A6 cells. Cells were incubated with either a negative control ascites (*Neg*) or mAbs specific for *CD80* (104) and *class II MHC* (AIMHCII), followed by a FITC-labeled secondary Ab

ved from this experiment, expression of CD80 and/or CD86 was similar or even higher compared with EBV-transformed human B lymphoblasts (M7) and was stable for at least 4 months of in vitro propagation. Subsequently, tumor cell variants were incubated with allogeneic peripheral blood mononuclear cells of healthy donors and T-cell proliferation was determined. Similar to the nontransfected SW480 cells, neither transfectant was capable of activating resting T lymphocytes. Moreover, T-cell activation was also not observed when T cells were cocultured with a mixture of CD80 and CD86-expressing SW480 cells or the CD80 and CD86-coexpressing variant (not shown).

CD54 and CD80

In the next set of experiments we addressed an additional difference between melanoma cells and colon cancer cells, namely expression of CD54, the ligand of CD11a/18. SW480 cells are negative for CD54, while SkMel63 cells express considerable levels of this cell-cell interaction molecule (Table 1). To this end, we transfected SW480 cells and the CD80-positive variant SW480A6 with a plasmid containing CD54 cDNA. Figure 6 shows an immu-

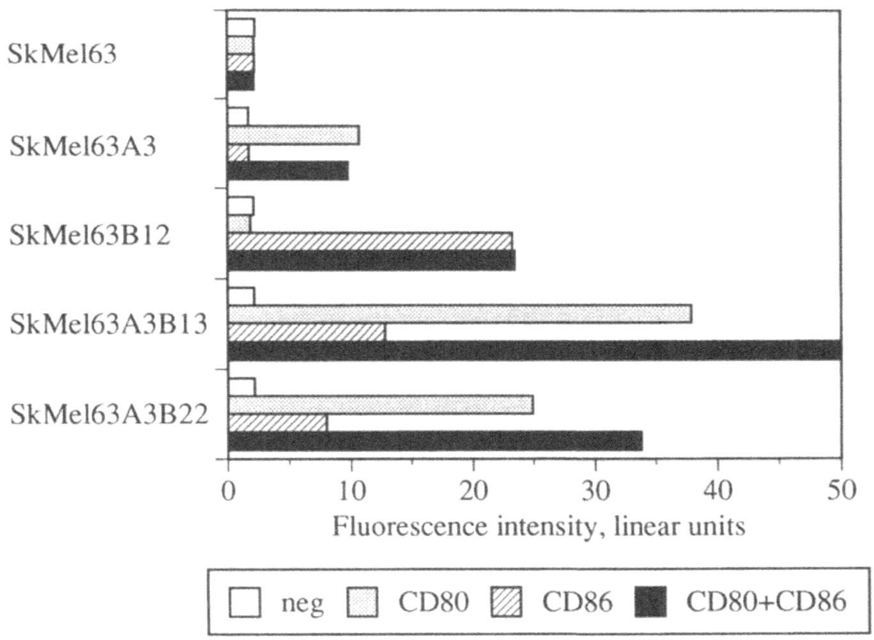

Fig. 5. Fluorescence analysis of CD80 and CD86-transfected SkMel63 sublines. Cells were incubated with either a negative control ascites (*neg*), the CD80-specific mAb 104 (*CD80*), the CD86-specific mAb IT2.2 (CD86), or a combination of both mAbs (*CD80 + CD86*) followed by a FITC-labeled secondary Ab. Fluorescence intensity represents mean values for each sample (5000 cells) on a linear scale

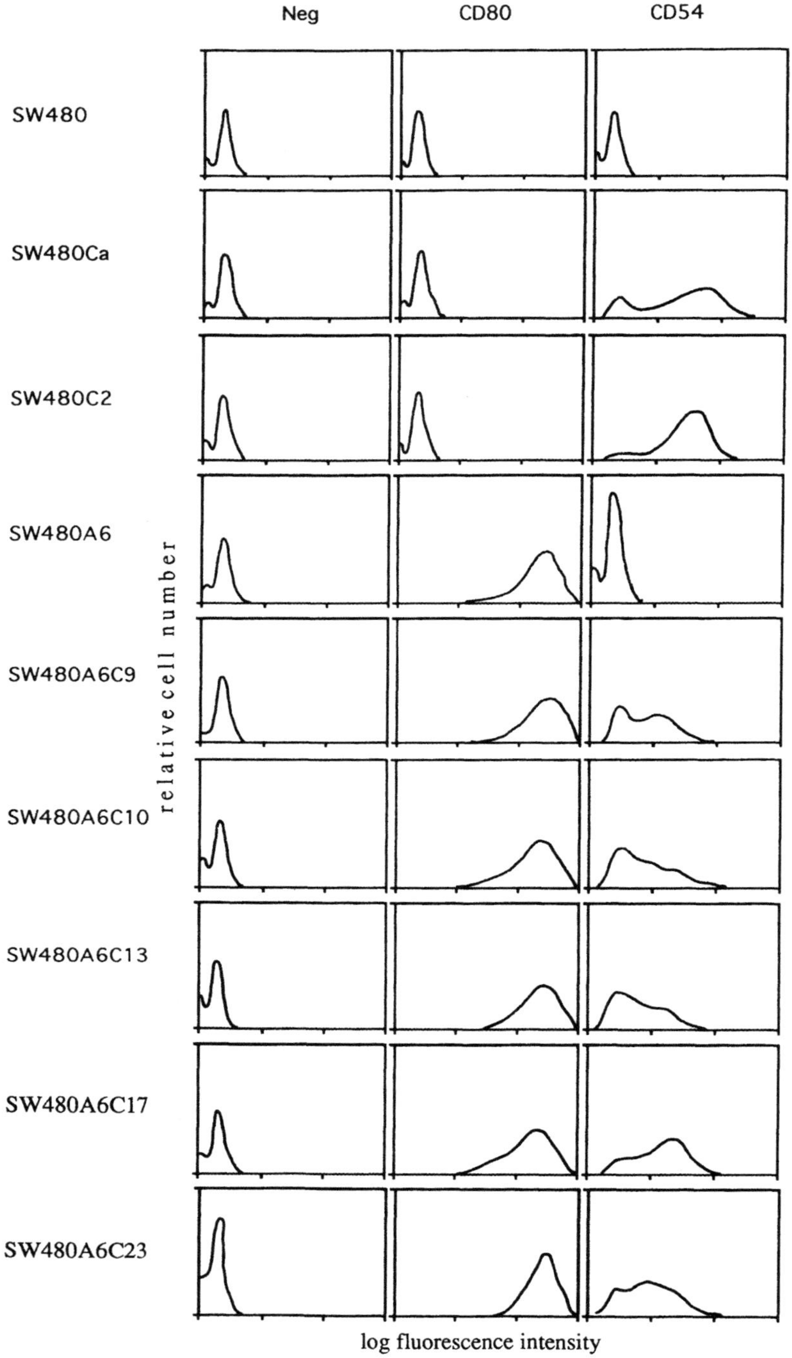

Fig. 6. Immunofluorescence of CD54-transfected SW480 and SW480A6 cells. Samples were incubated with a ngative control ascites (Neg) or mAbs specific for CD80 (104) or CD54 (MEM112), followed by a phycoerythrin-labeled secondary Ab

nofluorescence analysis of representative CD54c and CD54c/CD80c sublines. When these cells were investigated in MLTC, again no significant degree of T-cell proliferation was observed in a series of experiments. Although CD54 expression was rather low (compared with CD80 expression), variants coexpressing CD54 plus CD80 showed a strong costimulation which was up to five-fold higher than that of cells expressing CD80 only. However, this was only achieved in conjunction with submitogenic concentrations of OKT3.

CD54, CD80, and MHC Class II

The possibility remained that in order to induce T-cell activation, colon cancer cells such as SW480 require expression of at least three costimulation molecules, i.e., they have to express a phenotype which is similar to the phenotype of classic antigen-presenting cells (monocytes, macrophages, dentritic cells). To test this point, we selected SW480 cells transfected with CD80 and HLA-DR3 for variants which spontaneously express CD54. Such cells were enriched by sorting with magnetic beads. A phenotypic analysis of three variants derived in this system is shown in Fig. 7.

All three cell lines express CD80 at levels comparable to those of SW480A6. Moreover, a substantial fraction of cells express HLA-DR3 and CD54. When these variants were tested for their capacity to promote T-cell growth in vitro, strong proliferative responses of primary T cells were observed (Fig. 8). Moreover, it was possible to expand such T cells in the long term by weekly restimulation with tumor cell variants and by adding interleukin-2 following the third restimulation on day 17 in culture. Stimulation of T cells resulted in a continuous increase of CD8+ T cells and a decrease of CD4+ helper T cells. Importantly, CD8+ T-cell lines which were obtained under these experimental conditions were capable of lysing the nontransfected wild-type SW480 cells in a MHC-class-I-restricted fashion (as determined from the capacity of a class-I-specific monoclonal antibody to block cell-mediated lysis). In contrast, K562 cells (the standard target for natural killer cells) were not lysed. A monoclonal antibody capable of blocking MHC-class-II-restricted T-cell activity had no effect in this system. Nevertheless, one has to interpret the requirement of class II expression on immunogenic tumor cell lines as the requirement by CD8+ cytolytic preeffector cells of CD4+ T lymphocytes in order to differentiate into tumor-reactive killer cells.

Conclusions

We have tested the hypothesis that a major deficiency of tumor cells in their interaction with the host immune system is their inability to express adhe-

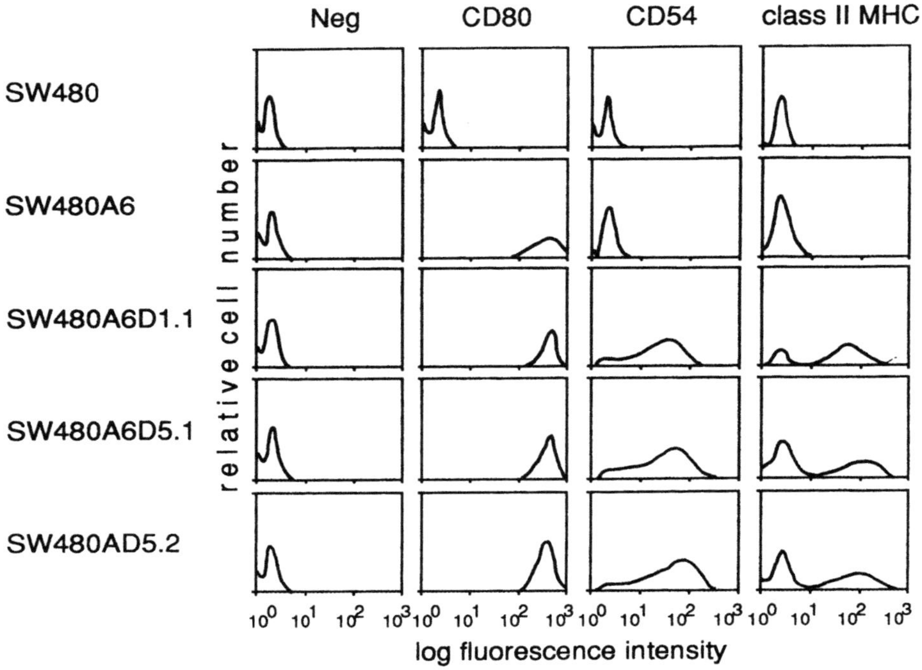

Fig. 7. Immunofluorescence of SW480 sublines. Cells were incubated with either a negative control ascites (*Neg*), the CD80-specific mAb 104 (*CD80*), the CD54 specific mAb MEM 112 (*CD54*), or MHC-class-II-specific mAb AIMHCII (*class II MHC*), followed by a FITC-labeled secondary phycoerythrin-labeled Ab

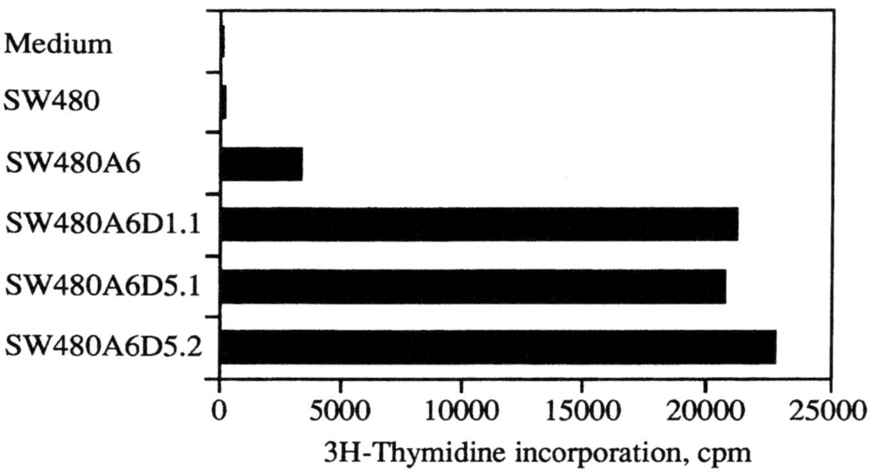

Fig. 8. T lymphocyte proliferative response toward SW480 variants: 10^5 resting peripheral blood T cells were incubated for 5 days with 10^4 irradiated SW480 colorectal cancer cell variants. Subsequently, cell proliferation was determined by ^{3}H-labeled thymidine incorporation

sion molecules known to provide costimulatory signals for lymphocyte activation. If this were the case, then rational strategies to improve the immunogenicity of tumor cells could be based on adhesion molecule expression by somatic gene transfer into tumor cells rather than substituting cytokines. The latter act at a much later state than the former in the well-orchestrated cascade of events underlying effector cell generation in the immune system. Costimulation is a critical requirement for activation of resting T lymphocytes.The absence of costimulation in the context of antigen recognition by the T-cell receptor has been identified as one efficient mechanism to produce T-cell tolerance through the induction of anergy or even apoptosis [1-3].

We have sequentially introduced several genes through stable plasmid transfection into non-immunogenic colon cancer cell lines. Subsequently, these cells were investigated for their capacity to activate resting human T lymphocytes in an allogeneic situation (MLTC). Our data allow the following conclusions to be made:

1. Expression of CD80 (the ligand of CD28) appears to be necessary although insufficient to produce T-cell activation in vitro. The same applies to CD54 and MHC class II antigen.
2. In the experimental system employed here, CD86 and CD80 do not produce detectable differential nor synergistic functional effects.
3. Colon cancer cells coexpressing CD54 and CD80 have a stronger costimulatory potential, but only in conjunction with a T-cell receptor stimulus (mitogenic CD3-antibody).
4. Importantly, SW480 cells expressing MHC class II antigen (DR3) together with CD54 and CD80 are capable of inducing T-cell proliferation. Such tumor cell variants could be employed to propagate human CD8+ T cells expressing MHC-class-I-restricted cytolytic activity in a long term culture.
5. Once activated, T effector lymphocytes are capable of killing nontransfected wild-type tumor cells. This demonstrates that differential requirements exist for the activation of resting preeffector cells and expression of effector function. While the former process appears to be highly regulated (which is likely to prevent autoaggression) the latter is of much lower stringency. This makes it feasible to employ genetically modified tumor cells for vaccination of tumor-bearing individuals with the expectation of generating tumor-reactive effector T cells that can eliminate unmodified malignant tissue.
6. Tumor cell variants such as those described here should allow the generation of colon-cancer-specific T cells with the perspective of identifying novel tissue or tumor-specific (target) antigens.

References

1. Van Seventer GA, Newman W, Shimizu Y, Nutman TB, Tanaka Y, Horgan KJ, Gopal TV, Ennis E, O'Sullivan D, Grey H, Shaw S (1991) Analysis of T cell stimulation by superantigen plus major histocompatibility complex class II molecules or by CD3 monoclonal antibody: costimulation by purified adhesion ligands VCAM-1, ICAM-1, but not ELAM-1. J Exp Med 174:901–916
2. Damle NK, Klussman P, Linsley PS, Aruffo A (1992) Differential costimulatory effects of adhesion molecules B7, ICAM-1, LFA-3, and VCAM-1 on resting and antigen-primed CD4+ T lymphocytes. J Immunol 148:1985–1990
3. Freeman G, Freedman AS, Segil JM, Lee G, Withman JF, Nadler LM (1989) B7, a member of the IG superfamily with unique expression on activated and neoplastic B cells. J Immunol 143:2714–2719
4. Gimmi CD, Freeman GJ, Gribben JG, Sugita K, Freedman AS, Morimoto C, Nadler LM (1991) B-cell surface antigen B7 provides a costimulatory signal that induces T cells to proliferate and secrete IL-2. Proc Natl Acad Sci USA 88:6575–6579
5. Norton SD, Zuckerman L, Uhrdahl KB, Shefner R, Miller J, Jenkins MK (1992) The CD28 ligand B7 enhances IL-2 production by providing costimulatory signals to T cells. J Immunol 149:1556–1561
6. Samstag Y, Eckerkorn C, Wesselborg S, Henning S, Wallich R, Meuer SC (1994) Costimulatory signals for human T cell activation induce the nuclear translocation of pp19/cofilin. Proc Natl Acad Sci USA 91:4494–4498
7. Schwarz RH (1990) A cell culture model for T lymphocyte clonal anergy. Science 248:1349–1356
8. Janeway CA Jr, Bottomly K (1994) Signals and signs for lymphocyte responses. Cell 76:275–278
9. Meuer SC, Hussey RE, Fabbi M, Fox D, Acuto O, Fitzgerald KA, Hodgdon JC, Protentis JP, Schlossman SF, Reinherz EL (1984) An alternative pathway of T cell activation: a functional role for the 50 KD T11 sheep erythrocyte receptor protein. Cell 36:897–906
10. Meuer SC, Schraven B, Samstag Y (1994) An alternative pathway of T cell activation. Int Arch Allergy Appl Immunol 104:216–221
11. Samstag Y, Dreizler EM, Ambach A, Sczakiel G, Meuer SC (1996) Inhibition of a constitutively active serine phosphatase in T lymphoma cells blocks nuclear translocation of pp19/cofilin and induces apoptosis. J Immunol 156:4167–4173
12. Schirren CA, Völpel H, Meuer SC (1992) Adhesion molecules on freshly recovered T leukemias promote tumor directed lympholysis. Blood 79:138–143
13. Archimbaud E, Thomas X, Campos L, Maguad JP, Dore JF, Fiere D (1992) Expression of surface adhesion molecule (CD54) ICAM-I and CD58 (LFA-3) in adult acute leukemia: relationship with initial characteristics and prognosis. Leukemia 6:265–271
14. Habicht A, Lindauer M, Galmbacher P, Rudy W, Gebert J, Schackert HK, Meuer SC, Moebius U (1995) Development of immunogenic colorectal cancer cell lines for vaccination: expression of CD80 (B7.1) is not sufficient to restore impaired primary T cell activation in vitro. Eur J Cancer 31A:2396–2402
15. Freeman GJ, Gribben JG, Boussiotis VA, Ng JW, Restivo VA, Lombard LA, Gray GS, Nadler LM (1993) Cloning of B7-2: a CTLA-4 counter-receptor that costimulates human T cell proliferation. Science 262:909–911
16. Azuma M, Ito D, Yagita H, Okomura K, Phillips JH, Lanier LL, Somoza C (1993) B70 antigen is a second ligand for CTLA4 and CD28. Nature 366:76–79
17. Hathcoek KS, Laszlo G, Dickler HB, Bradshaw J, Linsley P, Hodes RJ (1993) Identification of a CTLA-4 ligand costimulatory for T cell activation. Science 262:905–907

Gene-Modified Dendritic Cells as Vaccines for the Induction of Anti-Tumor Immunity

A. Pezzutto and J. Westermann

Introduction

In the last few years several laboratories have provided evidence that tumor-specific antigens can be defined by T lymphocytes in humans (Boon et al. 1994). These antigens have been identified mainly by cloning T lymphocytes that were isolated from peripheral blood or from tumor tissues (tumor-infiltrating lymphocytes). The restricted reactivity of the T-cell clones for specific alleles of the major histocompatibility complex (MHC) was a remarkably constant finding that was clarified and understood by the demonstration that small peptides can bind to the antigen-binding groove of molecules of the MHC. Intracellular proteins are degraded in the proteasomes into small peptides 8–14 amino acids in length, which are transported to the endoplasmic reticulum and loaded into the peptide-binding groove of newly synthesized MHC class I molecules. The MHC-peptide complexes are then exported on the cell membrane and presented to CD8 + T cells. It is now clear that tumor cells can also present autologous tissue-specific antigens. A number of molecules that are preferentially expressed in tumor cells have been identified in melanoma, renal cell carcinoma, breast cancer, ovarian and gastrointestinal cancer. The amino acid sequence of several peptides that interact with different MHC molecules has been defined in melanoma (Cox et al. 1994; Boon et al. 1994). However, most of these peptides are not strictly tumor-specific, being expressed either in normal melanocytes or in other tissues, such as testes or lung. Eliciting an immune reaction against these antigens may therefore induce autoimmunity: this is substantiated by the finding that melanoma patients responding to cytokine treatment frequently develop vitiligo. Other tumor-associated antigens that are currently being investigated as potential targets for immunotherapy approaches include oncogene products such as c-erb-B2 (HER-2/neo) (breast cancer) or ras (carcinomas, sarcomas, leukemias), products of "tumor suppressor genes" such as the p53 and Rb-1 genes that are deleted or mutated in different cancers, proteins derived from human papilloma viruses in cervical carcinoma, oncofetal proteins such as carcinoembrionic antigen (CEA), and altered mucins in breast and gastrointestinal cancer.

Symposium in Immunology VI
Eibl/Huber/Peter/Wahn (Eds.)

Lack of Immune Responsiveness against Tumors and Possible Ways of Restoring the Immunogenicity of Tumor Cells

If tumor-specific epitopes are indeed presented to the T-cell system in the context of the endogenous antigen presentation pathway, then the question arises why tumors develop at all in immunocompetent individuals. Probably several different mechanisms allow the tumors to escape immune surveillance, including defective antigen presentation and selective modulation of locally recruited T-cells. It is likely that both these mechanisms act synergistically to reduce antitumor immune responses. MHC class I molecules are downregulated in some tumors (Doyle et al. 1985; Elliot et al. 1989), either because the transcription of HLA class I α-chains is decreased, or because the binding of peptides to MHC molecules is impaired. Decreased synthesis of proteasome components and impaired synthesis of the TAP transporter proteins that regulate entry of peptide fragments into the endoplasmic reticulum have been demonstrated in some tumors (Restifo et al. 1993). On the other hand, inhibitory factors and cytokines can be secreted by the tumor to downmodulate the function of locally recruited T cells, such as transforming growth factor-β, IL-10, and other cytokines.

A further mechanism that may explain tolerance to tumor-associated antigens has been elucidated recently: T cells recognizing peptide-MHC complexes require additional signals in order to be properly activated. Only cells that coexpress accessory molecules on their surface – as do antigen-presenting cells – are able to trigger cytotoxic T-cell responses (Chen et al. 1993; Linsley and Ledbetter 1993). These accessory molecules stabilize adhesion between antigen-presenting cell and T cell and deliver activating signals to the T cell. Although many tumors do express MHC molecules, tumor cells do not bear costimulatory molecules, inducing tolerance rather than cytotoxic immunity. One of the strategies for the induction of antitumor immunity aims at modifying tumor cells to express costimulatory molecules. Poorly immunogenic tumor cells can be converted into cells capable of inducing potent immune response by transfecting the genes coding for the CD80 antigen B7-1 (Chen et al. 1992a, 1994; Townsend and Allison 1993; Dunussi-Joannopoulos et al. 1996). An important observation of these experiments was that, while the expression of CD80 was necessary for the generation of immunocompetent cells, it was not required in the "effector" phase of the cytotoxic reaction, for killing of untransfected tumor cells. Such strategies aimed at turning tumor cells into better antigen-presenting cells are currently being evaluated in gene therapy protocols.

Based on the background of the poor immunogenicity of tumor cells, a further strategy has been developed recently: instead of providing the tumor cell with antigen-presenting cell features, effective recognition of tumor-associated antigens is achieved by inducing expression of tumor epitopes on professional antigen-presenting cells. In this approach dendritic cells are either pulsed with a tumor-associated antigen or gene modified to constitutively express the antigen (Knight et al. 1985; Grabbe et al. 1991; Cohen et al. 1994; Flamand et al. 1994, Alijagic et al. 1995). Dendritic cells are potent antigen-presenting cells of bone marrow origin that play a crucial role in the initiation of MHC-restricted T-cell responses to foreign antigens, in particular for the priming of naive T cells (Inaba et al. 1987, Bhardwaj et al. 1994).

According to the conventional view on antigen presentation pathways, it was first believed that antigens loaded onto the surface of dendritic cells would be processed only along the extracellular pathway inducing MHC class II restricted responses (Fig. 1). Recently, however, Kovacsovic-Bankowsky and Rock (1995) have provided clear evidence that peptide pulsing in vitro may indeed lead to MHC class I-restricted CD8 responses (Fig. 1, gray pathway). Celluzzi et al. (1996) showed that dendritic cells pulsed with an ovalbumin peptide protected mice against a lethal challenge with a tumor cell line that had been transduced with ovalbumin. The protection was specific for ovalbumin and was mediated by CD8+ T cells. When the mice were challenged with the wild-type parental cell line they were also protected, suggesting that the antigen-presenting cells during the immune recognition of

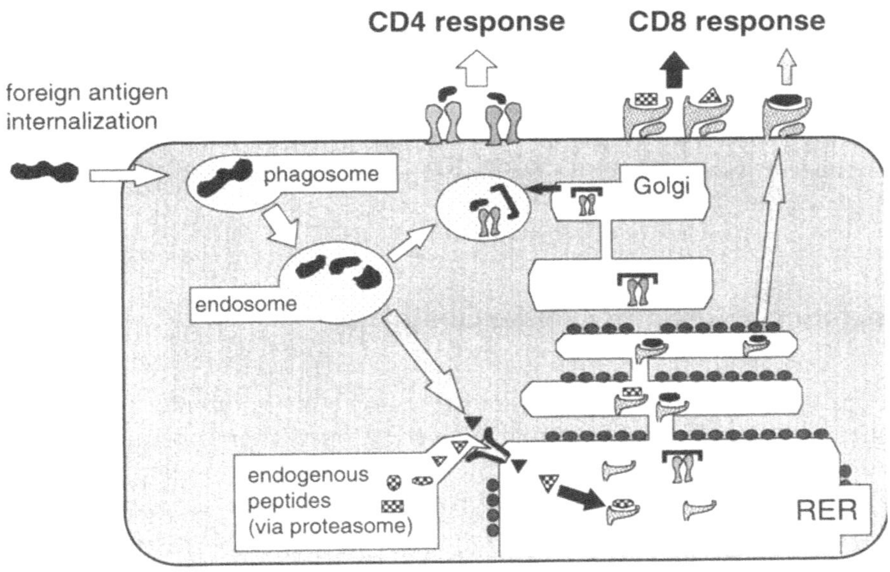

Fig. 1. Pathways of antigen presentation. Exogenous antigens that have been internalized and digested in endophagolysosomes interact with the peptide-binding groov of MHC class II molecules when the invariant chain is displaced in the acidic environment of transport vesicles. Intracytoplasmic proteins are digested to small peptides and transported to the endoplasmic reticulum (RER), where they interact with MHC class I molecules that are being synthesized. The MHC-peptide complexes are exported to the cell surface. The existence of a pathway that allows exogenous peptides to enter RER and load MHC class I molecules has been recently shown

ovalbumin had also acknowledged other tumor-specific antigens and induced protective immunity against them also. A remarkable finding was reported by Paglia et al. (1996), who showed that dendritic cells pulsed with an intact soluble antigen (β-galactosidase) could induce tumor protection against a tumor cell line that had been transduced with β-galactosidase. In this case also the cytotoxic response was mediated by CD8+ cytolytic T lymphocytes, demonstrating that the soluble protein had been processed and presented via MHC class I to T cells in vivo. Mayordomo et al. (1995) even demonstrated the therapeutic potential of tumor peptide-pulsed dendritic cells in animals with established tumors. Promising preliminary results have been recently described by Hsu et al. (1996), who were able to induce both measurable antitumor cellular responses and clinical improvement in lymphoma patients treated with dendritic cells pulsed with the idiotypic proteins of their lymphoma cells.

Although all these data demonstrate that dentritic cells can load exogenous peptides into their MHC class I molecules, targeting tumor-specific antigens to the cytosolic compartment of antigen-presenting cells using gene transfer techniques may still have some advantages in clinical settings: transfection would lead to cytoplasmic expression of different peptide fragments, among which the cell will ultimately select those fitting its own MHC molecules. Moreover, it is conceivable that inducing constitutive expression of an antigen in the antigen-presenting cell will result in a higher number of MHC molecules expressing the tumor epitope than will peptide loading: results, however, may vary in different experimental settings and with different antigens. Finally, gene transfer techniques may be used to insert cytokine genes to further improve the ability of dendritic cells to locally recruit and/or activate T cells.

Generation of Dendritic Cells for Clinical Use

In our laboratory dendritic cells are generated by two different techniques: purified CD34 cells from patients recovering from chemotherapy-induced bone marrow aplasia are cultured in the presence of granulocyte macrophage-colony stimulating factor (GM-CSF) and tumor necrosis factor-α (TNF-α) for 7 days and for a further 5 days in the presence of GM-CSF, TNF-α and IL-4. The addition of IL-4 to the culture represents a slight modification of the method described by Caux et al. (1992); GM-CSF is used at a concentration of 100 ng/ml, TNF-α is used at 10 ng/ml, and IL-4 is used at 1000 U/ml. Alternatively, dendritic cells can be generated from peripheral blood mononuclear cells as described by Romani et al. (1994) and Sallusto and Lanzavecchia (1994). Briefly, T and B cells are depleted using immunomagnetic beads, while the non-T-, non-B-cell population is cultured for 7 days at a density of 1×10^6 cells/ml in medium containing GM-CSF and

IL-4 at the concentrations indicated above. After 6–7 days of culture the cells are collected for analysis and functional experiments. Figure 2a shows the typical dendritic ("veiled") morphology of cells generated from T- and B-depleted peripheral blood mononuclear cells; Fig. 2b shows the electron microscopy analysis revealing the typical cytoplasmic extensions devoid of organelles, the abundance of mitochondria, and the scantiness of other intracytoplasmic organelles. Phenotypical features of dendritic cells are shown in Fig. 3: CD3, CD19, and CD14 antigens are negative, while MHC class I and class II antigens are expressed at high density, together with CD1a, CD80, CD86, and CD40. The myeloid antigens CD13 and CD33 are positive, as are several adhesion molecules including CD11a, b, c, CD44, and CD54.

Dendritic cells are strong stimulators in allogeneic and autologous mixed lymphocyte reaction. Compared to the non-T-cell fraction, which is enriched for B cells and monocytes, dendritic cells are up to 30-fold better stimulators of allogeneic responses: already at a stimulator to responder ratio of 1:312 (dendritic : T cells), significant T-cell proliferation occurs.

The bcr-abl Fusion Protein of Chronic Myeloid Leukemia is an Ideal Tumor-Specific Antigen

In our opinion, the fusion proteins that originate from the chromosomal translocations frequently found in hematological malignancies are particularly attractive as potential targets for tumor-directed immunotherapy because of their truly tumor-specific distribution. Translocation sites frequently involve genes coding for enzymes or regulatory proteins, resulting in functional abnormalities that are likely to be causally linked to the malignant behavior of the cells. Elimination of the cells expressing the translocation should eradicate the tumor, and downmodulation of antigen expression should not occur, allowing "escape" from immune surveillance.

In chronic myeloid leukemia (CML), malignant transformation occurs as the consequence of a reciprocal translocation between chromosomes 9 and 22, leading to an abnormal chromosome 22 with a shorter long arm (Philadelphia chromosome). This event transposes the c-abl proto-oncogene from its normal position on chromosome 9 to the breakpoint cluster region (bcr) of chromosome 22. The breakpoint on chromosome 9 always involves exon 2 (abl2 or "a2"), while the breakpoint on chromosome 22 may involve either exon 2 (bcr2 or "b2") or exon 3 (bcr3 or "b3"), resulting in either a "b3a2" or a "b2a2" new hybrid BCR-ABL oncogene (reviewed in Kantarijan et al. 1993). The fusions are always in frame and translate into new functional hybrid RNAs, which encode for new 210-kDa (p210) functional chimeric proteins that consist of either 1906 (b2a2) or 1931 (b3a2) amino acids. Both bcr-abl chimeric proteins have a similar, abnormally increased, tyrosine kinase activity which turns the affected hematopoietic progenitor cells into ab-

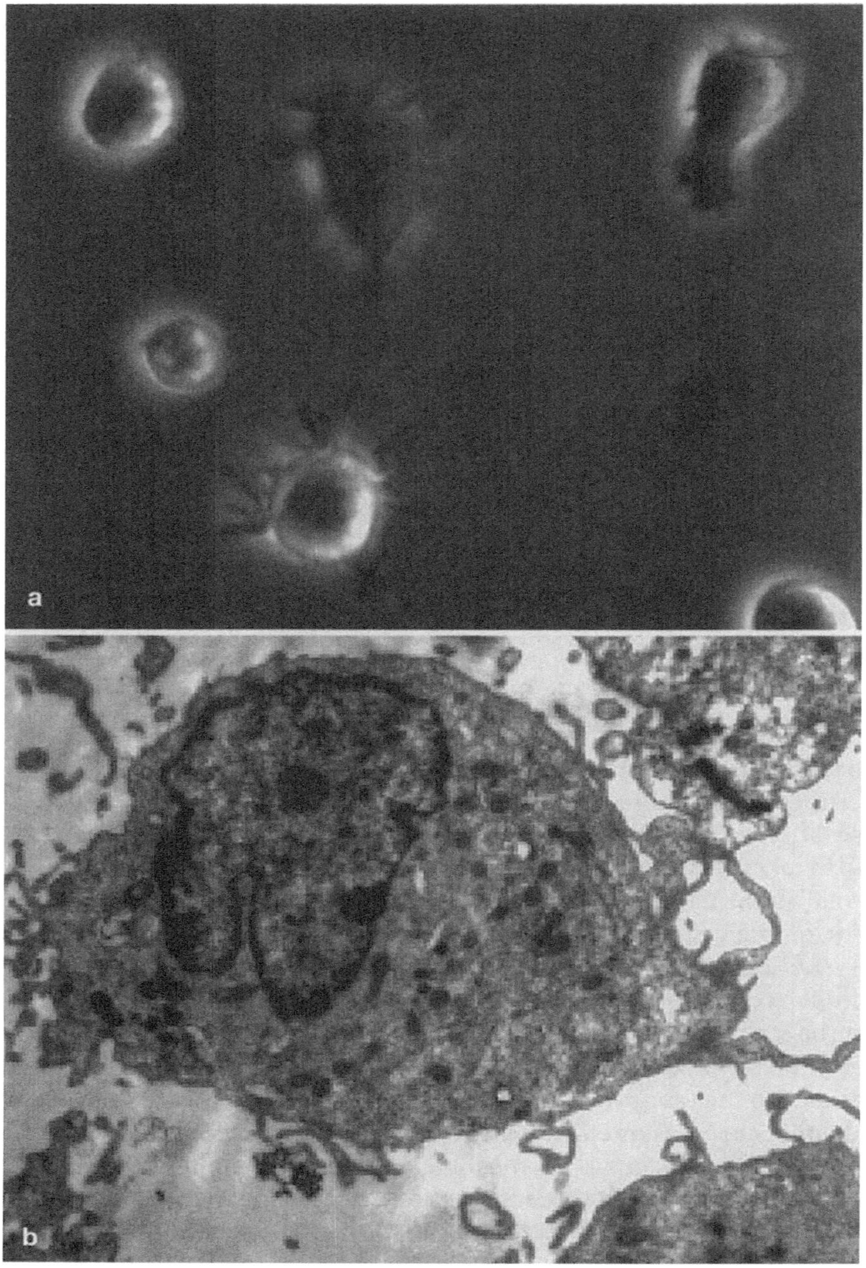

Fig. 2a. Contrast phase microscopy of dendritic cells generated from T- and B-cell-depleted mononuclear cells allows easy morphological identification. **b** Electron microscopy of the same preparation shows details of the cytoplasmic extensions, the abundance of mitochondria, and the paucity of other organelles

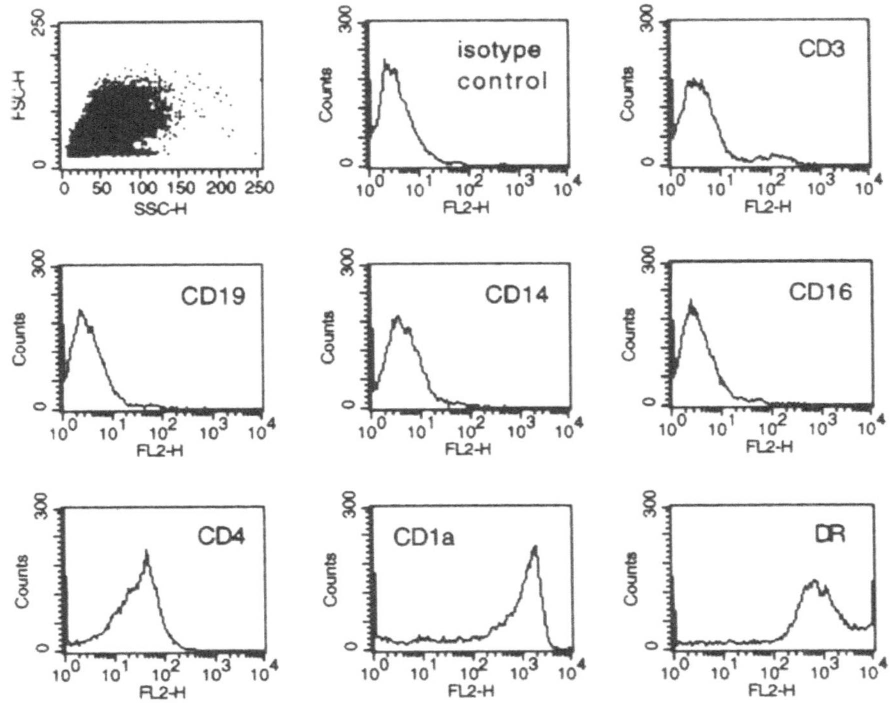

Fig. 3. Flow cytometry profile of dendritic cells generated from T- and B-cell-depleted mononuclear cells: T, B, and NK markers are absent, MHC molecules, myelomonocytic markers and adhesion and costimulatory molecules are highly upregulated. The expression of CD1a is typical of dendritic cells

normally proliferating cells. Since the transformation does not affect the ability of the progenitor cells to undergo differentiation, a whole progeny of blood cells bearing the chromosomal aberration is generated: bcr-abl-positive cells are widely found in the myeloid, monocytic, megakaryocytic, and B-cell lineages of the patients (Fig. 4).

Like any other intracellular component, the bcr-abl fusion protein also undergoes processing along the endogenous pathway of antigen presentation, so that immunogenic peptides of the protein are presented on the cell surface in the context of MHC class I molecules, where they could be eventually recognized by T cells (Chen et al. 1992b). While it must be assumed that peptides originating from the normal bcr and abl gene products are tolerated by the immune system during ontogeny, a peptide spanning the fusion region of bcr-abl should be recognized as new or "foreign" and elicit a T-cell response. Among all the different peptides that span the fusion region of bcr-abl, three peptides have been shown to bind to HLA-A3.2, HLA11, or HLA-B8 with high to intermediate affinity (Bocchia et al. 1995). Peptides

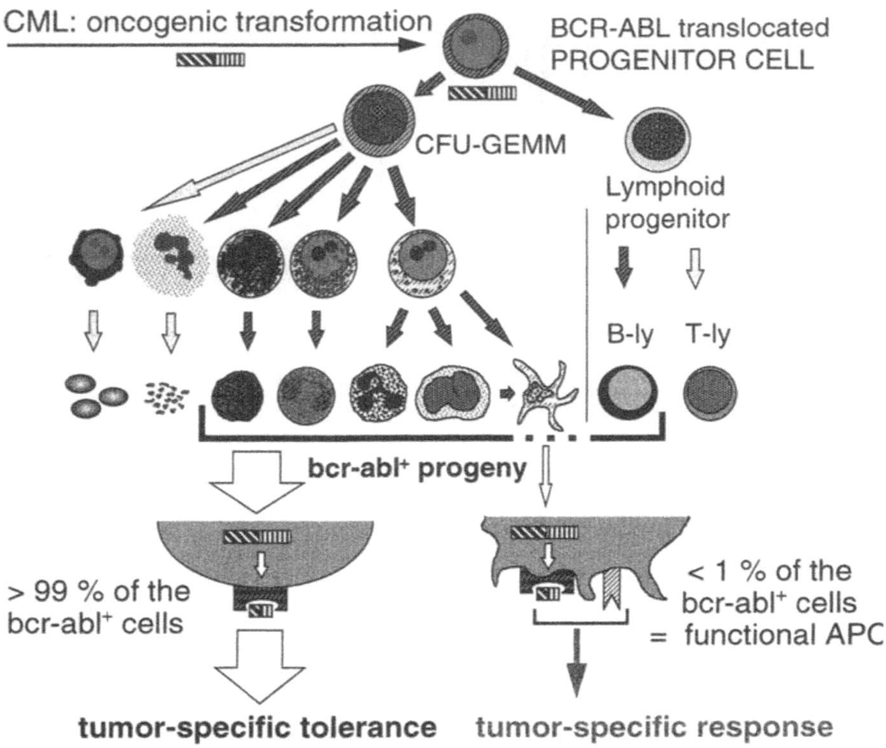

Fig. 4. In chronic myeloid leukemia the chromosomal translocation affects not only progenitor cells but also mature circulating leukocytes including dendritic cells. Disease-specific fusion peptides can be presented to T lymphocytes by MHC class I-expressing cells, but tolerance is likely to dominate over stimulation because of the lack of costimulatory molecules on the vast majority of the cells

ATGFKQSSK, KQSSKALQR, and HSATGFKQSSK bind to HLA-A11 and HLA-A3.2 while the peptide GFKQSSKAL binds to HLA-B8.

T-cell clones specific for bcr-abl peptides can be generated by pulsing dendritic cells of individuals with the appropriate HLA specificity in vitro; these T-cell clones specifically recognize CML cells (Bocchia et al. 1996). The clinical relevance of immunity to bcr-abl is further – albeit indirectly – supported by the observation first made by Kolb et al. (1990) that patients with CML in relapse after allogeneic bone marrow transplantation can be cured simply by transfusions of leukocytes from the same allogeneic donor. Although an immune response to foreign "minor" MHC antigens could at least partially explain this remarkable phenomenon, it is tempting to speculate that reactivity to bcr-abl plays a role in determining the specificity of the immune reaction (graft versus leukemia effect). Still, interferon can induce hematological remissions in about 20 % of CML patients: although the mechanism of action is far from being understood, the immunomodulatory activity of interferon – particularly the upregulation of MHC molecules – may contribute to its therapeutic activity.

Dendritic Cell-Based Approaches for the Treatment of CML

We have generated dendritic cells from both CD34+ progenitor cells and peripheral blood monocytes in patients with CML. With both techniques, cells with the typical morphological and phenotypical features of dendritic cells were generated. In functional experiments dendritic cells derived from CD34+ progenitor cells provided consistently stronger stimulation of normal allogeneic T cells than did dendritic cells generated from peripheral blood mononuclear cells.

Since dendritic cells originate from bone marrow progenitor cells, which are the target of the 9:22 chromosomal translocation in CML, it is likely that – according to disease stage – variable percentages dendritic cells express the 9:22 translocation, with almost 100 % positivity in the accelerated phase. In HLA A3-2+, HLA-A11+, and HLA-A8+ individuals, the tumor-specific bcr-abl fusion peptide should be expressed as processed peptide on the surface of CML cells. In this situation, even unmodified dendritic cells could provide a vaccination stimulus for the generation of bcr-abl-specific immunity. Since the large majority of CML cells, however, would express the bcr-abl fusion peptide but not the CD80 or CD86 costimulatory molecules necessary for the induction of specific immunity, peripheral tolerance is likely to be present in vivo (Fig. 4). For this reason, we tried to improve the immunogenicity of dendritic cells by transducing the gene coding for IL-7 into DC. IL-7 was chosen because in several cytokine transduction experiments it had a very strong immunostimulatory effect, increasing tumor immunogenicity in a T-cell-dependent way, thereby inducing tumor rejection (Hock et al. 1991; Aoki et al. 1992). Moreover, tumor cells transfected to coexpress CD80 and IL-7 were a very potent vaccine in a murine model (Cayeux et al. 1995). Finally, IL-7 has been shown to support the in vitro growth of $CD8^+$ CTLs for a prolonged period of time: the T cells maintained their antigenic specificity even without the continuous stimulation of antigen-presenting cells (Lynch and Miller 1994).

As a first step, we tested the feasibility of gene transfer in human dendritic cells using β-galactosidase as a reporter gene: dendritic cells can be efficiently transfected using the lac-Z retroviral vector. Transfection efficiencies of 40 %–55 % were consistently obtained by incubating dendritic cells with virus-containing supernatant and performing three sequential cycles of infection on days 2, 3, and 4 of the culture. Persistence of the bacterial DNA in dendritic cells was documented up to 20 days in culture (Aicher et al. 1996).

When the IL-7 vector was used, a higher variation in the amount of transfected cells was achieved: this was confirmed by measuring the amount of IL-7 secreted in cultures of dendritic cells, which ranged from 80 pg/ml up to >7000 pg/ml. IL-7-transfected dendritic cells were consistently more potent than unmodified dendritic cells in stimulating T-cell proliferation (Fig. 5). A vaccination protocoll that includes the administration of ex-vivo-generated, autologous dendritic cells to HLA-A3+, HLA-A11+, and HLA-B8+ patients with CML in the accelerated phase is currently planned at our institution. Future protocols will include the administration of gene-modified, IL-7 secreting dendritic cells to CML patients, possibly those with minimal residual disease.

Conclusions

Immunotherapy with dendritic cells is an attractive model for the treatment of several conditions, including infectious diseases and cancer. Both peptide

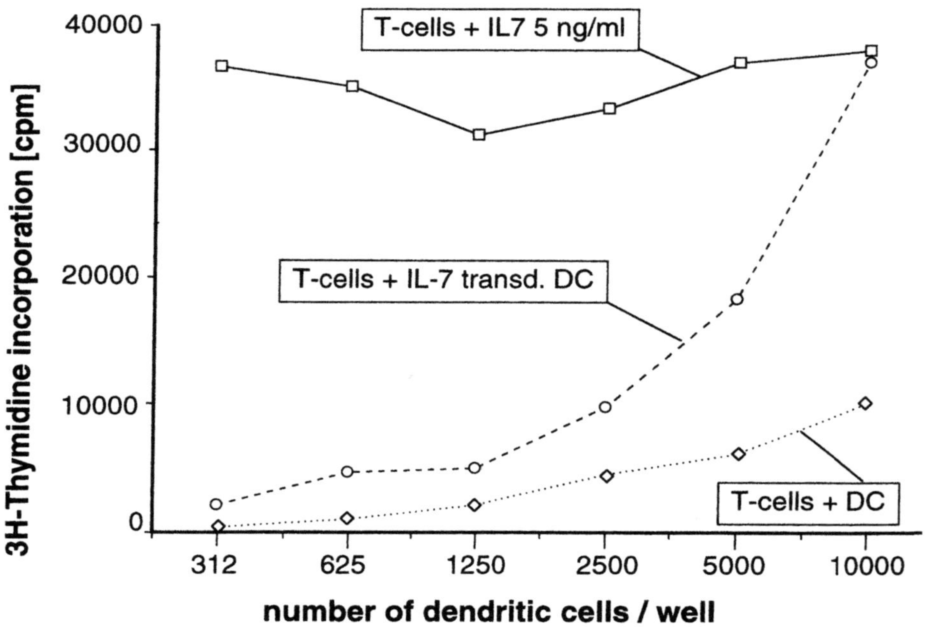

Fig. 5. Stimulatory effects of dendritic cells transfected with a retroviral vector coding for IL-7 in the presence of allogeneic T cells. 10^5 T cells were cultivated in the presence of scalar doses of dendritic cells. As controls, T cells were cultured in the presence of IL-7 at 5 ng/ml. In the culture wells with 10^4 dendritic cells, enough IL-7 is produced to equal the amount of T-cell proliferation observed in the presence of exogenous IL-7 at 5 ng/ml

pulsing and gene modification are feasible. Peptide-pulsed dendritic cells could be used when the tumor epitopes of a given antigen are known and MHC restriction has been defined; gene-modified dendritic cells might be useful when the MHC-relevant epitopes of tumor-associated antigens have not yet been defined. Gene modification may also improve the function of dendritic cells, helping to overcome any existing tolerance.

In CML dendritic cells already express the relevant tumor antigen: in our opinion this disease represents an ideal clinical setting for the evaluation of dendritic cell-based vaccination in cancer.

References

Aicher A, Westermann J, Cayeux S, Daemen K, Willimsky G, Uckert W, Blankenstein Th, Dörken B, Pezzutto A (1996) Successful retroviral transduction of a reporter gene in human dendritic cells: feasibility of therapy with gene-modified antigen presenting cells. Exp Hematol in press

Alijagic S, Möller P, Artuc M, Jurgovsky K, Czarnetzki BM, Schadendorf D (1995) Dendritic cells generated from peripheral blood transfected with human tyrosinase induce specific T cell activation. Eur J Immunol 25:3100–3107

Aoki T, Tashiro K, Miyatake S, Kinashi T, Nakano T, Oda Y, Kikuchi H, Honjo T (1992) Expression of murine interleukin-7 in a murine glioma cell line results in reduced tumorigenicity in vivo. Proc Natl Acad Sci USA 89:3850–3854

Bhardwaj N, Bender A, Gonzalez N, Bui LK, Garrett MC, Steinman RM (1994) Influenza virus-infected dendritic cells stimulate strong proliferative and cytolytic responses from human CD8+ T cells. J Clin Invest 94:797–807

Bocchia M, Wentworth PA, Southwood S, Sidney J, McGraw K, Scheinberg DA, Sette A (1995) Specific binding of leukemia oncogene fusion protein peptides to HLA class I molecules. Blood 85:2680–2684

Bocchia M, Korontsvit Z, Xu Q, Mackinnon S, Yang SY, Sette A, Scheinberg DA (1996) Specific human cellular immunity to bcr-abl oncogene-derived peptides. Blood 87:3587–3592

Boon T, Cerottini JC, Van den Eynde B, van der Bruggen P, Van Pel A (1994) Tumor antigens recognized by T lymphocytes. Annu Rev Immunol 12:337–365

Caux C, Dezutter-Dambuyant C, Schmitt D, Banchereau J (1992) GM-CSF and TNF-α cooperate in the generation of dendritic Langerhans cells. Nature 360:258–261

Cayeux S, Beck C, Aicher A, Dörken B, Blankenstein T (1995) Tumor cells cotransfected with interleukin-7 and B7-1 genes induce CD25 and CD28 on tumor infiltrating T lymphocytes and are strong vaccines. Eur J Immunol 25:2325–2331

Celluzzi Ch M, Mayordomo JI, Storkus WJ, Lotze MT, Falo Jr LD (1996) Peptide-pulsed dendritic cells induce antigen-specific, CTL-mediated protective tumor immunity. J Exp Med 183:283–287

Chen L, Ashe S, Brady WA, Helrström I, Hellström KE, Ledbetter JA, McGowan P, Linsley P (1992a) Costimulation of antitumor immunity by the B7 counterreceptor for the T lymphocyte molecules CD28 and CTLA-4. Cell 71:1093–1099

Chen W, Peace DJ, Rovira DK, You SG, Cheever MA (1992b) T-cell immunity to the joining region of $p210^{BCR-ABL}$ protein. Proc Natl Acad Sci 89:1468–1472

Chen L, Linsley PS, Hellström KE (1993) Costimulation of T cells for tumor immunity. Immunol Today 14:483–486

Chen L, Mc Gowan P, Ashe S, Johnston JV, Hellström I, Hellström KE (1994) B7-1/CD80 transduced tumor cells elicit better systemic immunity than wild-type tumor cells admixed with Corynebacterium parvum. Cancer Res 54:5420–5428
Cohen PhJ, Cohen PA, Rosenberg St A, Katz St I, Mulé JJ (1994) Murine epidermal Langerhans cells and splenic dendritic cells present tumor-associated antigens to primed T cells. Eur J Immunol 24:315–319
Cox AL, Skipper J, Chen Y, Henderson RA, Darrow TL, Shabanowitz J, Engelhard VH, Hunt DF, Slingluff Jr CL (1994) Identification of a peptide recognized by five melanoma-specific human cytotoxic T cell lines. Science 264:716–719
Doyle A, Martin WJ, Funa K, Gazdar A, Carney D, Martin SE, Linnoila I, Cuttitta F, Mulshine J, Bunn P, Minna J (1985) Markedly decreased expression of class I histocompatibility antigens, protein and mRNA in human small-cell lung cancer. J Exp Med 161:1135–1141
Dunussi-Joannopoulos K, Weinstein HJ, Nickerson PW, Strom TB, Burakoff SJ, Croop JM, Arcece RJ (1996) Irradiated B7-1 transduced primary acute myelogenous leukemia (AML) cells can be used as therapeutic vaccines in murine AML. Blood 87:2938–2946
Elliot BE, Carlow DA, Rodricks A, Wade A (1989) Perspectives on the role of MHC antigens in normal and malignant cell development. Adv Cancer Res 53:181–187
Flamand V, Sornasse T, Thielemans K, Demanet C, Bakkus M, Bazin H, Tielemans F, Leo O, Urbain J, Moser M (1994) Murine dendritic cells pulsed in vitro with tumor antigen induce tumor resistance in vivo. Eur J Immunol 24:605–610
Grabbe S, Bruvers B, Gallo RL, Knisely TL, Nazareno R, Granstein RD (1991) Tumor antigen presentation by murine epidermal cells. J Immunol 146:3656–3661
Hock H, Dorsch M, Diamantstein T, Blankenstein T (1991) Interleukin 7 induces CD4+ T cell dependent tumor rejection. J Exp Med 174:1291–1298
Hsu FJ, Benike C, Fagnoni F, Liles TM, Czerwinski D, Taidi B, Engelman EG, Levy R (1996) Vaccination of patients with B-cell lymphoma using autologous antigen-pulsed dendritic cells. Nature Medicine 2:52–58
Inaba K, Young JW, Steinman RM (1987) Direct activation of CD8+ cytotoxic T lymphocytes by dendritic cells. J Exp Med 166:182–194
Inaba K, Metlay JP, Crowley MT, Steinman RM (1990) Dendritic cells pulsed with protein antigens in vitro can prime antigen-specific, MHC-restricted T cells in situ. J Exp Med 172:631–640
Kantarijan HM, Deisseroth A, Kurzrock R, Esterov Y, Talpaz M (1993) Chronic myelogenous leukemia: a concise update. Blood 82:691–703
Knight SC, Hunt R, Dore C, Medawar PB (1985) Influence of dendritic cells on tumor growth. Proc Natl Acad Sci USA 82:4495–4497
Kolb HJ, Mittermüller J, Clemm C, Holler E, Ledderose G, Brehm G, Heim M, Wilmanns W (1990) Donor leukocyte transfusions for treatment of recurrent chronic myelogenous leukemia in marrow transplant patients. Blood 76: 2462–2470
Kovacsovics-Bankowski M, Rock KL (1995) A phagosome-to-cytosol pathway for exogenous antigens presented on MHC class I molecules. Science 267:243–245
Linsley PS, Ledbetter JA (1993) The role of the CD28 receptor during T cell responses to antigen. Annu Rev Immunol 11:191–212
Lynch DH, Miller RE (1994) Interleukin 7 promotes long-term in vitro growth of antitumor cyptotoxic T lymphocytes with immunotherapeutic efficacy in vivo. J Exp Med 179:31–42
Mayordomo JI, Zorina T, Storkus WJ, Zitvogel L, Celluzzi C, Falo LD, Melief CJ, Ilstad ST, Kast WM, Deleo AB, Lotze MT (1995) Bone marrow-derived dendritic cells pulsed with synthetic tumour peptides elicit protective and therapeutic anti-tumour immunity. Nature Medicine 1:1297–1302

Paglia P, Chiodoni C, Rodolfo M, Colombo MP (1996) Murine dendritic cells loaded in vitro with soluble protein prime cytotoxic T lymphocytes against tumor antigen in vivo. J Exp Med 183:317–322
Restifo NP, Esquivel F, Kawakami Y, Yewdell JW, Mulé JJ, Rosenberg SA, Bennink JR (1993) Identification of human cancers deficient in antigen processing. J Exp Med 177:265–272
Romani N, Gruner St, Brang D, Kämpgen E, Lenz A, Trockenbacher B, Konwalinka G, Fritsch PO, Steinman RM, Schuler G (1994) Proliferating dendritic cell progenitors in human blood. J Exp Med 180:83–93
Sallusto F, Lanzavecchia A (1994) Efficient presentation of soluble antigen by cultured human dendritic cells is maintained by granulocyte/macrophage colony-stimulating factor plus interleukin 4 and downregulated by tumor necrosis factor a. J Exp Med 179:1109–1118
Townsend SE, Allison JP (1993) Tumor rejection after direct costimulation of CD8+ T cells by B7-transfected melanoma cells. Science 259:368–371
Zitvogel L, Mayordomo JI, Tjandrawan T, DeLeo AB, Clarke MR, Lotze MT, Storkus WJ (1996) Therapy of murine tumors with tumor peptide-pulsed dendritic cells: dependence on T cells, B7 costimulation, and T helper cell 1-associated cytokines. J Exp Med 183:87–97

Potent Presentation of Soluble Protein Antigens by In Vitro-Generated Dendritic Cells from Peripheral Blood CD34$^+$ Progenitor Cells

B. Herbst, P. Fisch, A. Mackensen, G. Köhler, G. Wolff-Vorbeck, F. M. Rosenthal, H. Veelken, R. Mertelsmann, and A. Lindemann

Introduction

Dendritic cells (DC) are potent antigen-presenting cells (APC) and thus are specifically involved in the initiation of antigen-specific immune responses. Due to their potent costimulatory activity, they are well suited to prime naive T cells to various antigens (Ag), such as viral peptides, tumor-, or allo-antigens. In line with their crucial role in the host defense system, they are located in the epithelial borders of the body, where they take up Ag and then migrate into the lymph nodes to recruit T cells [1]. DCs originate from hematopoietic progenitor cells, and it has been shown recently that they can be generated from cord blood and peripheral blood progenitor cells (PBPC) in vitro by using granulocyte-macrophage colony-stimulating factor (GM-CSF) in conjunction with interleukin-4 (IL-4; [3]) or tumor necrosis factor-α (TNF–α; [2]). By adding GM-CSF and IL-4 to a combination of early acting hematopoietic growth factors we observed a ten-fold increase in the number of DCs derived from CD34$^+$ PBPCs compared with GM-CSF plus IL-4 or TNF-α alone [3]. In addition, large numbers of Birbeck-granule-positive "Langerhans-like" cells (LC) which are thought to be the immediate precursors of mature DCs, emerged under these conditions. Here we have analyzed the functional capacity of these cells to take up, process, and present a soluble protein antigen.

Materials and Methods

Media and Reagents

Cells were cultured in RPMI 1640 supplemented with 200 mmol/l L-glutamine, 50 μ*M* β-mercapthoethanol, 100 m*M* sodium pyruvate, 50 μg/ml streptomycin, 50 U/ml penicillin, MEM vitamins, and 10% FCS (56°C for 0.5 h; Boehringer Mannheim, Mannheim, Germany). The following recombinant human cytokines werde used: IL-1β, IL-3, GM-CSF, IL-4, and stem cell factor (SCF), all from Genyme Corp., Cambridge, MA; IL-6 (kindly provided by L. Färber, Sandoz AG, Nürnberg, Germany); erythropoietin (EPO; Cilag, Bad

Symposium in Immunology VI
Eibl/Huber/Peter/Wahn (Eds.)

Homburg, Germany). Human recombinant cytokines were used at a concentration of 10 ng/ml (IL-1β, SCF), 50 ng/ml (IL-4), 100 ng/ml (IL-3, IL-6) and 1 U/ml (EPO).

Mobilization of PBPCs and $CD34^+$ Selection

Patients received two cycles of conventional dose VP16, ifosfamide, cisplatin (VIP), with or without epirubicin (VIP-E) at three weekly intervals [4]. Granulocyte colony-stimulation factor (G-CSF; Neupogen, Amgen, Basel, Swizerland) was administered to all patients at a dose of 5 µg/kg per day s.c., in order to prevent chemotherapy-associated neutropenia and to mobilize PBPCs following chemotherapy [5]. Mobilized PBPCs were harvested by leukapheresis on day 10 or 11 after the second cycle of chemotherapy [5]. The $CD34^+$ progenitor cells were positively selected using the Ceprate avidin-biotin immunoadsorption column (Cellpro, Bothell, WA, USA), as described [5].

Culture of DCs from $CD34^+$ PBPCs

The method for the in vitro culture of human DCs has been described [3]. Briefly, the culture of purified $CD34^+$ cells was performed in 6-well-plates (Flacon, Heidelberg, Germany) in supplemented RPMI/10 % FCS in the presence of IL-1β, IL-3, IL-6, SCF, EPO (SE136), IL-4, and GM-CSF. Culture medium was replenished weekly. Cells were seeded at a concentration of 5×10^4 cells/ml at the beginning of culture, at a concentration of 5×10^5/ml in the second week, and at a concentration of 1×10^6 cells/ml thereafter. On day 24 cells were harvested and used for experiments.

Flow Cytometric Analysis and Cell Sorting

Surface marker analysis of in vitro cultured cells was performed using a FACScan (Becton Dickinson) and the Lysis II software. Monoclonal antibodies conjugated to FITC or phycoerythrin for direct fluorescence included anti-CD1a (Coulter Immunology, Hialeah, FL), CD36, CD40, CD54, CD58, CD23 (all from Immunotech, Marseille, France), CD14, HLA-DR, and CD80 (all from Becton-Dickinson & Co., Mountain View, CA). Cell sorting of subpopulations was performed on a FACStar Plus cell sorter (Becton Dickinson).

Antigen Presentation Assay with Autologous Antigen-Specific T Cells

Heparinized blood samples were collected prior to chemotherapy, and peripheral blood leukocytes (PBL) were isolated on Ficoll gradients. Antigen-reactive T cells from each patient were generated essentially as described [6]. In brief, PBLs were primed for seven days in RPMI 1640 medium, supplemented with 10 % human serum, antibiotics, L-glutamine and 10 m*M* HEPES buffer, containing tetanus toxoid (TT) at a concentration of 200 µg/ml (kindly provided by Dr. Blackolb, Behring, Marburg, Germany). On day 7, rhIL-2 (25 U/ml) was added to the soluble-antigen-primed T cells that were then expanded for additional 3 days before cryopreservation in aliquots. Antigen-primed T cells were thawed 2 days prior to the antigen presentation experiments and cultured in medium containing IL-2 (25 U/ml). Following in vitro culture of LCs/DCs from $CD34^+$ PBPCs, the cells were irradiated (40 Gy), washed, and used as APCs for the autologous TT-primed T cells. The assay was performed in 96-well flat-bottomed plates with a final volume of 200 µl/well. APCs were serially diluted and 3×10^4/well responder T cells and TT antigen were added as appropriate. The plates were incubated for 48 h at 37 °C, 5 % CO_2. Subsequently, the cells were pulsed with ^3H thymidine (1 µCi/well), incubated overnight, harvested on filters and counted by liquid scintillation as described [4, 5].

Results

Leukapheresis products were obtained from patients after chemotherapy and G-CSF treatment at the time of hematopoietic cell recovery and used as a starting material to purify $CD34^+$ PBPCs. These cells were positively selected to a purity of 70 %–95 % by an avidin immunoaffinity column [5]. The cells were $CD34^+CD1a^-$ (Fig. 1A). After 24 days in culture in the presence of SE136, GM-CSF and IL-4 a major population of large cells with high granularity (side scatter) had emerged that was strongly positive for CD1a while being $CD34^-$ [Fig. 1A, region 1 (R1)]. By electron microscopy, the majority of the $CD1a^{++}$ cells contained Birbeck granules [3], thus resembling typical Langerhans cells, the presumed precursor of mature CDs. The cells in R1 were analyzed further for expression of markers of known importance for APCs. They were found to express molecules involved in Ag uptake such as the low-affinity IgE-receptor CD23 and CD36, a molecule that is involved in phagocytosis [7]. Also, high expression of MHC class II molecules for Ag presentation was detected, as well as the presence of adhesion molecules CD54 (intercellular adhesion molecule-1) and CD58 (lymphocyte function associated antigen-3), and costimulatory molecules CD80 (B7-1) and CD86 (B7-2, not shown).

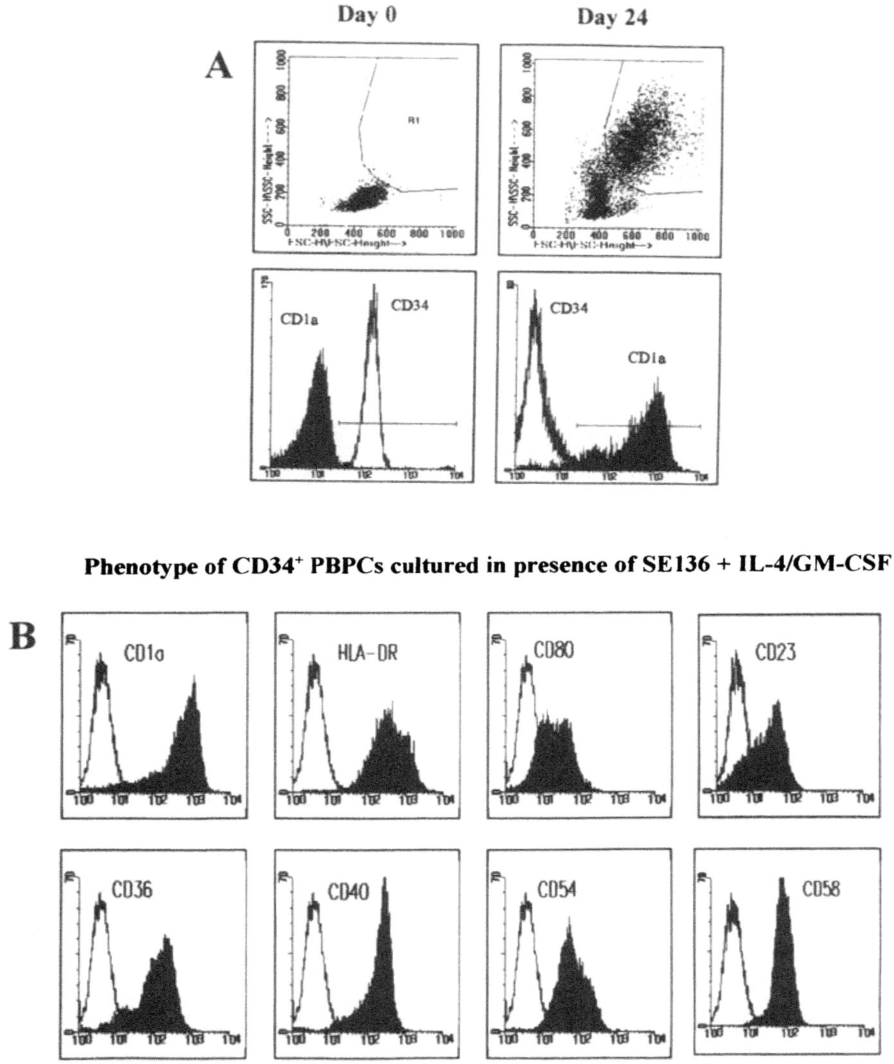

Fig. 1A, B. Flow cytometric analysis of in vitro-generated DCs from peripheral blood $CD34^+$ progenitor cells. **A** CD34+ PBPCs (*day 0*) were $CD1a^-$ (see *histogram, ungated cells*). Culture of these cells in the presence of SE136, IL-4 and GM-CSF for 24 days led to the generation of very large (forward scatter, FSC) cells with high granularity (side scatter, SSC; *day 24*). These cells were $CD34^-CD1a^{++/+}$ (see *histogram, cells gated in R1*). **B** Surface phenotype of $CD34^+$ PBPC-derived DCs (*R1* in **A**) cultured for 24 days in medium containing SE136, IL-4, and GM-CSF. The filled histograms represent the staining for the specific surface antigen, while the empty overlaid histograms represent the isotype controls

In order to analyze the antigen-presenting function of these cells, freshly separated $CD34^+$ cells and those cultured for 24 days under the conditions described above were tested for their ability to present the soluble antigen tetanus toxoid (TT) to autologous TT-specific T cells. These T cells had been primed in vitro to TT and were antigen specific (data not shown). In the absence of APCs there was little if any response of the primed T cells, indicating that processing of the TT and/or costimulation by the APCs was necessary for effective T cell stimulation (Fig. 2). Also, there was no T cell re-

A

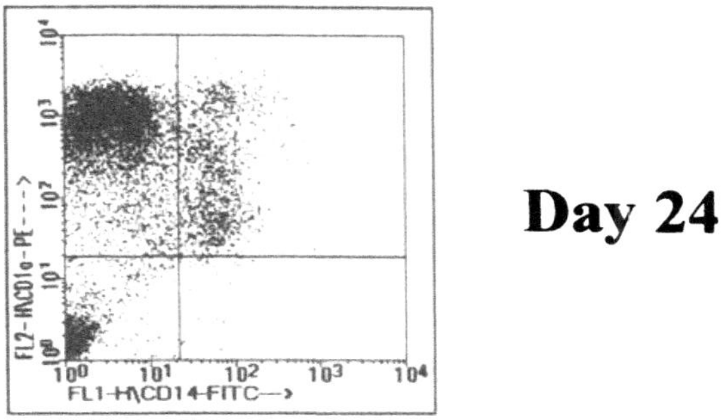

B

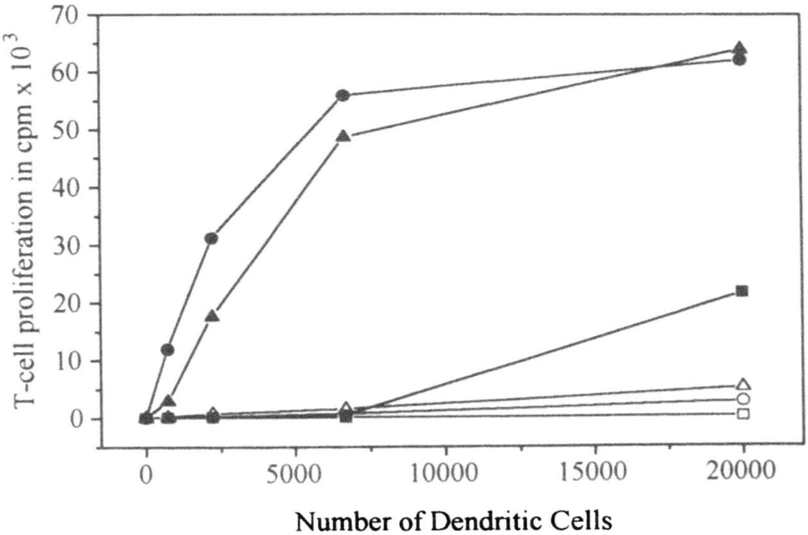

Fig. 2 Presentation of soluble TT by in-vitro-cultured DCs to autologous TT-specific T cells **A** The dot plot shows surface expression of CD1a (FL-2) and CD14 (FL-1) by day 24 of culture. Three subpopulations ($CD1a^+/CD14^-$, $CD1a^+/CD14^+$ and $CD1a^-/CD14^-$) were sorted and used as APCs in antigen presentation assays. **B** TT-specific T cells were incubated with different numbers of autologous APCs from "day 24"-cultures sorted as described in **A** in the presence (*filled symbols*) and absence (*open symbols*) of TT Ag. *Circles* represent $CD1a^+CD14^-$, triangles represent $CD1a^+CD14^+$, and *squares* represent $CD1a^-CD14^-$. The results shown are means of triplicate determinations with SD being less than 15% of the mean

sponse to the irradiated APCs in the absence of the antigen (data not shown). However, in the presence of both APCs and TT we observed vigorous proliferation of the primed T cells (Fig. 2). By titrating the number of APCs, we found that these APCs were very potent, with less than 750 APCs per microwell giving detectable responses. Half-maximal responses were observed with about 2500 APCs per well. Freshly purified $CD34^+$ cells were non-functional as APCs in this assay [8]. Since some of the $CD1a^+$ cells coexpressed CD14, we isolated $CD1a^+CD14^-$ cells and $CD1a^+CD14^+$ cells by FACS and compared them in the functional assays. As shown in Fig. 2, both subpopulations of these DCs were equally potent APCs of soluble TT antigen. $CD1a^-CD14^+$ cells were not generated under these culture conditions at sufficient amounts to be studied separately for APC function.

Discussion

Dendritic cells and macrophages function as professional APCs of exogenous antigens that require antigen uptake, processing, and presentation. After phagocytosis, micro-, or macropinocytosis [9], the antigen enters the endocytic pathway where it is degraded by proteases resulting in the production of the antigenic peptides. Generally, such peptides derived from exogenous antigens associate with MHC class II molecules in an as yet poorly defined compartment, which may be the MIIC structures [10], before being transported to the cell surface [11] where they can stimulate naive or primed T cells of the $CD4^+$ T cell subset.

While cultured macrophages have been described as being incapable of effective uptake and presentation of soluble proteins and peptides [1], DCs derived from monocytes in the presence of IL-4 and GM-CSF were found to be extremely potent in this respect [11]. So far it is not known if Birbeck-granule-positive DCs that emerge from $CD34^+$ PBPCs may function as potent APCs also. By using early acting hematopoietic growth factors in conjunction with IL-4 as an inducer of differentiation and GM-CSF as a "survival factor", we were able to generate large numbers of these cells from PBPCs. As demonstrated in Fig. 2, these cells were highly potent APCs for the soluble protein antigen TT that requires Ag uptake, processing, and presentation. A subpopulation of the $CD1a^+$ cells which coexpressed CD14 exhibited similar APC function. Since the mean CD1a expression was lower on the $CD14^+$ cells, these might represent a more mature DC-type cell, similar to DCs derived from LCs, that downregulate CD1a expression. However, the exact nature of these $CD1a^+CD14^+$ cells remains to be defined.

The autologous TT-specific T cells proliferated in response to TT presented by few APCs but not to TT or APCs alone, and were therefore immunologically similar to TT-specific T cell clones. Half-maximal stimulation of these cells was achieved with about 2500 APCs per well which is in a range similar to that described for monocyte-derived DCs [11].

Given that more than 10^7 CD1a$^+$ cells can be generated from 10^6 CD34$^+$ cells [3] in these patients, our approach provides a suitable source of large numbers of potent APCs that may be useful clinically. By loading these cells with peptides or proteins derived from infectious agents or tumor tissue, or by transfection with the respective genes, specific T cells may be generated in vitro and by adoptive transfer also in vivo.

References

1. Steinman RM (1991) The dendritic cell system and its role in immunogenicity. Annu Rev Immunol 9:271
2. Caux C, Dezutter-Dambuyant C, Schmitt D, Banchereau J (1992) GM-CSF and TNF-α cooperate in the generation of dendritic Langerhans cells. Nature 360:258
3. Mackensen A, Herbst B, Köhler G, Wolff-Vorbeck G, Rosenthal FM, Veelken H, Kulmburg P, Schäfer HE, Mertelsmann R, Lindemann A (1995) Delineation of the dendritic cell lineage by generating large numbers of Birbeck granule-positive Langerhans cells from human peripheral blood progenitor cells in vitro. Blood 86:2699–2707
4. Brugger W, Frisch J, Schulz G, Mertelsmann R, Kanz L (1992) Sequential administration of interleukin-3 and granulocyte-macrophage colony-stimulating factor following standard-dose combination chemotherapy with etoposide, ifosfamide, and cisplatin, J Clin Oncol 10:1452
5. Brugger W, Birken R, Bertz H, Hecht T, Fisch J, Schulz G, Mertelsmann R, Kanz L (1993) Peripheral blood progenitor cells mobilized by chemotherapy plus granulocyte-colony stimulating factor accelerate both neutrophil and platelet recovery after high-dose VP16, ifosfamide and cisplatin. Br J Haematol 84:402
6. Chen BP, DeMars R, Sondel PM (1987) Presentation of soluble antigen to human T cells by products of multiple HLA-linked loci: analysis of antigen presentation by a panel of cloned, autologous, HLA-mutant Epstein-Barr virus-transformed lymphoblastoid cell lines. Hum Immunol 18:75
7. Ren Y, Silverstein RL, Allen J, Savill J (1995) CD36 gene transfer confers capacity for phagocytosis of cells undergoing apoptosis. J Exp Med 181:1857
8. Fisch P, Köhler G, Garbe A, Herbst B, Wider D, Schaefer HE, Brugger W, Mertelsmann R, Kanz L (1996) Ex vivo generation of antigen presenting cells for soluble protein antigens from peripheral blood CD34$^+$ hematopoietic progenitor cells in cancer patients. Eur J Immunol 26:595–600
9. Sallusto F, Cella M, Daniele C, Lanzavecchia A (1995) Dendritic cells use macropinocytosis and the mannose receptor to concentrate macromolecules in the major histocompatibility complex class II compartment: downregulation by cytokines and bacterial products. J Exp Med 182:389
10. Nijman HW, Kleijmeer MJ, Ossevoort MA, Oorschot VMT, Vierboom MPM, van de Keur M, Kenemans P, Kast WM, Geuze HJ, Melief CJM (1995) Antigen capture and major histocompatibility class II compartments of freshly isolated and cultured human blood dendritic cells. J Exp Med 182:163
11. Sallusto F, Lanzavecchia A (1994) Efficient presentation of soluble antigen by cultured human dendritic cells is maintained by granulocyte/macrophage colony-stimulating factor plus interleukin 4 and downregulated by tumor necrosis factor α. J Exp Med 179:1109

Interleukin-12: Biology and Clinical Studies

W. E. Aulitzky and C. Huber

Introduction

The communication of the various components of the immune system is controlled by the interaction of soluble and cell-bound molecules. This coordinate function of immune cells is critical for the successfull defense against viral, bacterial, and parasitic pathogens. Moreover, defects of the immune system are also involved in the pathogenesis of malignant and autoimmune disease. The innate immune system, in particular the phagocyte system, represents the first line of defense against infectious pathogens. Soluble products produced by phagocytic cells after contact with invading microbes recruit T cells to the site of the infectious invasion. This leads to induction of an antigen-specific immune response and aids the sucessful clearing of the invading pathogen.

Interleukin-12 (IL-12) is one of the cytokines produced during the early phase of the immune response by phagocytic cells and plays a critical role for the induction of an antigen-specific cellular immune response. IL-12 was discovered in 1989 by two independent groups; one group described it as a natural killer (NK) cell stimulatory factor and, the other described it as a lymphocyte maturation factor (Kobayashi et al. 1989; Stern et al. 1990). Subsequent cloning revealed the molecular identity of these two cytokines (Gubler et al. 1991; Wolf et al. 1991; Schoenhaut et al. 1992). IL-12 induces cytokine secretion by T cells and NK cells and acts as a growth factor for T cells and NK cells (Trinchieri 1995; Trembleau et al. 1995).

Biochemistry of Human IL-12 and the Human IL-12 receptor

The biochemical structure of IL-12 is different from that of most other cytokines described so far (Kobayashi et al. 1989; Stern et al, 1990; Hirao et al. 1995; Gubler et al. 1991). The active molecule is a heterodimer consisting of two covalently linked polypeptide chains with molecular weights of 35 kDa (p35) and 40 kDa (p40; Table 1). The RNA of p35 encodes a 219 amino acid polypeptide with a predicted molecular weight of 27.5 kDa. The p35 peptide contains seven cysteine residues and three potential N-glycosylation sites.

Symposium in Immunology VI
Eibl/Huber/Peter/Wahn (Eds.)

Table 1 Biochemistry of IL-12. (See text for abbreviations)

	p35	p40
Number of amino acids	219	328
Predicted molecular weight	27.5 kDa	34.7 kDa
Carbohydrate content	20%	10%
Chromosome location	3p12–13.2	5q31–33
Homology (mouse/human)	70%	60%
Homology (to other proteins)	IL-6, G-CSF	IL-6 receptor, G-CSF-receptor

Twenty percent of the natural product consists of carbohydrates (Podlask et al. 1992). Comparison of the murine and human p35 sequence shows a homology in the range of 60% (Schoenhaut et al. 1992). The gene coding for p35 is located on chromosome 3p12–3p13.2 (Sieburth et al. 1992). The primary structure of the p35 protein suggests the formation of four alpha helices. The p35 protein displays a significant homology with granulocyte colony-stimulating factor (G-CSF) and IL-6 (Merberg et al. 1992).

The p40 cDNA sequence codes for a 328 amino acid chain with a 22 amino acid signal sequence. The mature protein has a calculated molecular weight of 34.7 kDa with ten cysteine residues, four N-glycosylation sites, and a carbohydrate content of 10 % (Podlaski et al. 1992). The p40 gene has been mapped to chomosome 5q31–5q33 (Sieburth et al. 1992). IL-12 p40 is not homologous to any other cytokine, however, the protein shows significant homology to the extracellular part of several members of the hematopoietic cytokine receptor family (Schoenhaut et al. 1992; Gearing and Cosman 1991). The molecule contains four cysteine residues in conserved positions and a WSEWAS sequence, which is similar to the WSXWS consensus motif characteristic for this receptor family (Taga and Kishimoto 1993). The highest homology exists to the receptors for IL-6, G-CSF, and neurotrophic factor receptor alpha chain (CNTF-Rα). Interestingly, soluble forms of all of these receptors have been described. Moreover, in contrast to the antagonistic action of most soluble receptors, two of these soluble receptors (IL-6, CNTF-Rα) are capable of transmitting the cytokine signal via another membrane molecule (Taga and Kishimoto 1993). Thus, it appears that IL-12 has irreversibly captured its agonistic soluble receptor by covalent binding. The hypothesis of a common evolutionary origin of the IL-12 and the IL-6/CNTF cytokine–cytokine–receptor systems is further supported by the observation that both cloned IL-12 receptors are homologous to the signal transducing protein of the receptor system gp 130 (Chua et al. 1994). Murine IL-12 is active on both mouse and human cells (Schoenhaut et al. 1992). In contrast, the activity of human IL-12 is species specific. The species specificity is determined by the p35 protein.

Three different binding sites for IL-12 with affinities of 5-20 p*M*, 50–200 p*M*, and 2–6 n*M* have been identified on human cells (Desai et al. 1992; Chizzonite et al. 1992). Two receptor chains have been cloned and designated IL-12-receptor beta1 and beta2 (Chua et al. 1994). Both show significant homology with the gp130 signal transducing protein of the IL-6 receptor system (U. Gubler, data presented at the Meeting of the New York Academy of Sciences, November 1995). IL-12 receptors are found predominantly on activated T cells and NK cells (Desai et al. 1992). IL-12 binding leads to phosphorylation of the tyrosine kinases TYK2 and JAK2 (Bacon et al. 1995a). The signal is then transmitted to the nucleus by the STAT4 protein (Bacon et al. 1995b; Jacobson et al. 1995). Thus, IL-12 has a different signal transduction pathway than IL-2 which transmits its signal via phosphorylation of the kinases JAK 1 and JAK3.

Cell Sources and Regulation of IL-12 Synthesis

IL-12 has been cloned from Epstein-Barr virus (EBV)-transformed cell lines and the majority of these cell lines produce IL-12 (Schoenhaut et al. 1992; Wolf et al. 1991). In the peripheral blood, monocytes and neutrophils are the major source of IL-12. In addition, B cells, mast cells, dendritic cells, keratinocytes, and macrophages are a major source of IL-12 (D'Andrea et al. 1992; Gately 1993; Macatonia et al. 1995; Aragane et al. 1994; Muller et al. 1994).

The regulation of IL-12 synthesis is complex. Coordinate expression of both p35 and p40 in a cell is required for the production of bioactive IL-12. RNA for p35 is constitutively expressed in many different cell types, although no measurable quantities of isolated p35 can be detected (D'Andrea et al. 1992). RNA of p40 is found exclusively in cells capable of producing IL-12. The expression of both p35 and p40 can be induced, although the expression of p40 is increased to a much larger extent than the expression of p35 (Schoenhaut et al. 1992; D'Andrea et al. 1993; Wolf et al. 1991). Accordingly, cells producing IL-12 secrete a more than a ten-fold excess of p40 in comparison with p35. The physiological role for free p40 is not clear. In murine systems an antagonistic activity has been reported (Mattner et al. 1993). However, this is not the case for the human protein.

Peripheral blood mononuclear cells (PBMNCs) produce small amounts of IL-12 constitutively (D'Andrea et al. 1992; D'Andrea et al. 1993). However, this low constitutive production disappeared when the cells were cultured under endotoxin-free conditions. Microbial components are the most powerful stimuli for IL-12 production. LPS, fixed *Staphylococcus aureus*, streptococci, and mycobacteria have been shown to enhance the synthesis of IL-12 by PBMNCs (Kubin et al. 1994a; D'Andrea et al. 1992, Chehimi et al. 1994). In addition to regulation by pathogen-derived molecules, IL-12 release is regulated by a variety of cytokines. Interferon gamma (IFN-γ) and granulocyte-macrophage colony-stimulating factor (GM-CSF) induce the production of IL-12 (Kubin et al. 1994a). Direct interaction of T cells and monocytes via the CD40–CD40 ligand system is also capable of inducing the production of IL-12 (Shu et al. 1995). IL-12 production is reduced by IL-4, IL-10, transforming growth factor-beta and prostaglandin E2 (D'Andrea et al. 1993; van der Pouw Kraan et al. 1995).

In Vitro Studies with IL-12

Modulation of T-Cell Function by IL-12

IL-12 is a potent costimulator of T-cell proliferation. Whereas IL-12 has little mitogenic effect on resting T cells, the IL-2-, CD3-, phytohemagglutinin-, and alloantigen-induced proliferation of T cells is enhanced by IL-12 after several days of culture (Gately et al. 1991; Perussia et al. 1992). In addition, IL-12 is a mitogen for preactivated T cells and NK cells. The kinetics of this response is concurrent with the appearance of high affinity binding sites on the target cells (Desai et al.1992). The major target subpopulation of T cells for IL- 12 action is the CD30-positive T lymphocytes (Alzona et al. 1995). Both cytokine production and proliferation is preferentially induced in this cell type.

IL-12 promotes the development of T helper type 1 (TH-1) cell generation and antagonizes the activity of IL4, the major promoter of TH-2 responses (Manetti et al. 1993; Manetti et al. 1994; Wu et al. 1993). Addition of IL-12 to human T cells generates a TH1 pattern of cytokine production, i.e., cell clones producing high amounts of IFN-γ. Hence, blocking endogenously produced IL-12 with antibodies induces clones with a TH-2-like phenotype. This critical role of IL-2 for the development of the TH-1 type of the T-cell response has been confirmed in various antigen-dependent T-cell systems.

Regulation of NK Cell Function by IL-12

The proliferation of preactivated NK cells is enhanced by IL-12 (Gately et al. 1991; Perussia et al. 1992). In addition, IL-12 enhances the cytotoxicity of NK cells (Robertson et al. 1992). Although the maximum enhancement induced by IL-12 is clearly lower than after stimulation with IL-1 or IFN-α, the effective concentrations of IL-12 are much lower than effective concentrations of IL-2 or IFN-α (Chehimi et al. 1992; Rabinowich et al. 1993). IL-12 stimulates the synthesis of a variety of proteins involved in the cytotoxic attack of NK cells such as granzyme A and B or perforin (Aste Amezaga et al. 1994; Cesano et al. 1993; Salcedo et al. 1993).

Induction of Cytokines by IL-12

IL-12 is a potent inducer of a variety of cytokines in T cells and NK cells (Stern et al. 1990; Wolf et al 1991; Chan et al. 1991; Perussia et al. 1992; Kubin et al. 1994b; Aste Amezaga et al. 1994; Naume et al. 1993). Similar to IL-2, IL-12 enhances the synthesis of INF-γ, tumor necrosis factor-alpha (TNF-α), GM-CSF, M-CSF, IL-3, IL-8, and IL-2. The most relevant function is most likely the induction of IFN-γ. IL-12 is the most potent inducer of IFN-γ known so far and is clearly required for maximum production of this cytokine (Chan et al. 1991). In contrast to the other stimulatory effects on T cells and NK cells, IL-12 induces IFN-γ secretion also by resting T cells and NK cells. Cofactors for IL-12-induced IFN-γ production are TNF-α and IL-1β. In addition, stimuli mediated via the CD28–B7 system act synergistically with IL-12 (Gajewski et al. 1995; Kubin et al. 1994b). In summary, maximal stimulation of IFN-γ production by T cells is observed when three signals are delivered to the T cell: (1) stimulation of the T-cell receptor–CD3 complex; (2) stimulation of the B7–CD28 pathway; and (3) the soluble phagocyte-derived factor IL-12.

Extralymphatic Effects of IL-12

The growth of hematopoietic progenitor cells stimulated by FLT-3, stem cell factor, and IL-3 is enhanced by addition of IL-12 (Hirao et al. 1995; Jacobsen et al. 1993, Jacobsen et al. 1995; Bellone and Trinchieri 1994). This activity is at least partly dependent on the presence of accessory cells in the culture system (Bertolini et al. 1995). In vivo, the stimulatory effects of IL-12 on hematopoiesis are masked by antiproliferative activities of cytokines induced by IL-12 such as IFN-γ or TNF-α (Tare et al. 1995; Eng et al. 1995). An anti-angiogenic activity described for IL-12 also depends on the induction of IFN-γ (Voest et al. 1995, see comments).

Activity of IL-12 in Animal Models

Malignant Disease Models

Antitumor activity of IL-12 has been demonstrated in a variety of murine disease models. The mechanism of the antitumor activity of IL-12 has been studied in detail using the RENCA kidney cancer model. IL-12 cures the majority of mice; this effect is dependent on the presence of CD-positive T cells. In addition, the antitumor activity can be blocked by IFN-γ antibodies. However, IFN-γ administration is clearly less effective than IL-12 (Brunda et al. 1995). Thus, the antitumor activity of IL-12 is not solely caused by IFN-γ induction. Coadministration of low doses of IL-2 and IL-12 was synergistic in the RENCA and in a colorectal tumor model (Leder et al. 1995). In addition to direct antitumor effects, IL-12 might also be a potent adjuvant for vaccines against tumor-associated antigens (Noguchi et al.1995).

Infectious Disease Models

IL-12 is an essential component for the induction of a protective immune response to a variety of bacterial, viral, and parasitic infectious pathogens. IL-12 is produced during infection with bacteria and parasites, e.g., *Listeria monocytogenes* and *Toxoplasma gondii* (Vieira et al. 1994; Heinzel et al. 1994; Gazzinelli et al. 1994). Treatment with IL-12 is beneficial in a variety of infectious disease models.

Treatment with IL-12 both before and and after challenge with bacteria reduces the mortality of mice infected with group A streptococci (Metzger et al. 1995). IL-12 decreases the number of viable bacteria in mice inoculated with *Mycobacterium avium* (Kobayashi et al. 1995; Saunders et al. 1995). Mortality of mice is reduced by IL-12 in a variety of fungal infection models such as histoplasma and cryptococci (Zhou et al. 1995; Clemons et al. 1994). However, IL-12 might also contribute to the pathology of infection. Blocking IL-12 protects BCG-primed mice from LPS-induced death (Wysocka et al. 1995). Similarily, IL-12 has been identified as one of the key molecules mediating the pathology of the generalized Shwartzman reaction (Ozmen et al. 1994).

Endogenous IL-12 production is essential for mounting a protective TH1 response against leishmania (Ghalib et al. 1995; Heinzel et al. 1995). In addition to its protective role for certain parasites when administered before infection, IL-12 is an effective treatment also for established infection with leishmania (Heinzel et al. 1993; Murray and Hariprashad 1995). Mice treated with an anti-IL-12 antibody are unable to clear *T. gondii* (Hunter et al. 1995).

Only few virus models have been studied so far. Mice treated with IL-12 recover more quickly from infection with vesicular stomatitis virus (Bi et al. 1995). Unexpectedly, only minor beneficial effects were observed after treatment with low doses of IL-12 in murine cytomegalovirus and lymphocyte choriomeningitis virus infection, whereas high doses inhibited development of virus-specific CD8 + cytotoxic T lymphocytes (Orange et al. 1994; Orange et al. 1995b; Orange et al. 1995a). However, IL- 12 is capable of modulating the type of immune response to viruses. Recombinant adenoviruses used for gene therapy applications induce a TH-2 response causing the production of high titers of neutralizing IgA antibodies. This neutralizing immune response blocks the virus after the second administration and thereby limits the applicability of gene therapy using these vectors. IL-12 blocks the generation of these neutralizing antibodies in vivo (Yang et al. 1995, see comments). This might represent a strategy to successfully overcome one of the major obstacles of successful gene therapy.

Autoimmune Disease Models

IL-12 is involved in the protection from autoimmune disease caused by a TH-2 type immune response on the one hand and in the pathogenesis of TH-1 type diseases on the other hand. Administration of IL-12 with collagen type II induces a severe arthritis in mice (Germann et al. 1995). IL-12 enhances the sensitivity to contact allergens in mouse models (Maguire 1995; Muller et al. 1995). Antibodies to IL-12 abrogate established experimental colitis in mice (Neurath et al. 1995). In contrast, the development of TH-2-dependent diseases may be blocked by IL-12. Airway hyperresponsiveness, a pathophysiological hallmark of allergic asthma, is reduced by IL-12 (Gavett et al. 1995).

Preclinical Pharmacology of IL-12

IL-12 is a molecule with a molecular weight of 75 kDa. Therefore it should be the first cytokine which is not rapidly eliminated via the kidneys. This has been confirmed in rhesus monkeys treated with 42.5 µg/kg IL-12 either i.v. or s.c. (Nadeau et al. 1995). The compound was eliminated with kinetics compatible with a two-compartment model with a t1/2 lambda 1 ranging from 0.2 to 5 h and a t1/2 lambda 2 ranging from 13 to 19 h. The major proportion (85 %) of the dose was eliminated in the lambda 2 phase. Hence, the clearance rate was rather slow with 3 ml per h/kg after i.v. injection. After s.c. injection the peak concentration was reached 18 h after injection, and the bioavailability was in the range of 20 %–30 %. Although the pharmacokinetics may be different in humans, it seems likely that the pharmacokinetics of IL-12 is fundamentally different from that of other cytokines.

Clinical Studies

Two IL-12 preparations are presently in clinical development. Intravenous application of IL-12 have been tested in a phase I without major problems, but severe treatment associated toxic events including two treatment-related deaths have been observed in the first phase II trial (Cohen 1995). Although this discrepancy between the toxicities observed in the phase I and phase II trials has not been fully clarified, a minor change in the schedule of IL-12 is considered to be the reason for the increase in toxicity. Whereas the phase I trial was started with a test dose, the phase II trial immediately started with i.v. infusion for 5 days.

Two collaborative ongoing phase I trials with IL-12 (Roche) in Mainz, Rotterdam, Memorial Sloan Kettering and the Cleveland Clinic are testing the safety and pharmacodynamics of s.c. administration once weekly and three times weekly. No severe irreversible treatment-related adverse events have been observed so far with this compound. Dose-dependent fever and transient depression of leukocyte counts were observed in the majority of patients. In addition, mild elevations of liver function tests were observed. Dose-dependent induction of β-microglobulin and neopterin were observed indicating significant biological activity of IL-12 at the low doses used. These biological responses were observed at doses with minimal toxicity. No maximum tolerable dose has been defined and both trials are still ongoing.

Conclusion

IL-12 is a cytokine with unique biological and pharmacological properties. It is most potent for the treatment of a variety of malignant and infectious diseases in animal models. In some of these models IL-12 is clearly superior to other cytokines tested. In addition, the unique pharmacological profile with a prolonged serum half-life may allow the continuous exposure of patients to the cytokine. Preliminary results of clinical trials demonstrate that IL-12 (Roche) applied subcutaneously is a highly biologically active compound at doses with a minimal toxicity. The experience of the Genetics Institute, Johannes Gutenberg University, Mainz with i.v. application, however, should lead to a cautious clinical approach to further explore the therapeutic potential of this compound.

References

Alzona M, Jack HM, Fisher RI, Ellis TM (1995) IL-12 activates IFN-gamma production through the preferential activation of CD30+ T cells. J Immunol 154:9–16

Aragane Y, Riemann H, Bhardwaj RS, Schwarz A, Sawada Y, Yamada H, Luger TA, Kubin M, Trinchieri G, Schwarz T (1994) IL-12 is expressed and released by human keratinocytes and epidermoid carcinoma cell lines. J Immunol 153:5366–5372

Aste Amezaga M, D'Andrea A, Kubin M, Trinchieri G (1994) Cooperation of natural killer cell stimulatory factor/interleukin-12 with other stimuli in the induction of cytokines and cytotoxic cell-associated molecules in human T and NK cells. Cell Immunol 156:480–492

Bacon CM, McVicar DW, Ortaldo JR, Rees RC, O'Shea JJ, Johnston JA (1995a) Interleukin 12 (IL-12) induces tyrosine phosphorylation of JAK2 and TYK2: differential use of Janus family tyrosine kinases by IL-2 and IL-12. J Exp Med 181:399–404

Bacon CM, Petricoin EF 3rd, Ortaldo JR, Rees RC, Larner AC, Johnston JA, O'Shea JJ (1995b) Interleukin 12 induces tyrosine phosphorylation and activation of STAT4 in human lymphocytes. Proc Natl Acad Sci USA 92:7307–7311

Bellone G, Trinchieri G (1994) Dual stimulatory and inhibitory effect of NK cell stimulatory factor/IL-12 on human hematopoiesis. J Immunol 153: 930–937

Bertolini F, Soligo D, Lazzari L, Corsini C., Servida F, Sirchia G (1995) The effect of interleukin-12 in ex-vivo expansion of human haemopoietic progenitors. Br J Haematol 90: 935–938

Bi Z, Quandt P, Komatsu T, Barna M, Reiss CS (1995) IL-12 promotes enhanced recovery from vesicular stomatitis virus infection of the central nervous system. J Immunol 155: 5684–5689

Brunda MJ, Luistro L, Hendrzak JA, Fountoulakis M, Garotta G, Gately MK (1995) Role of interferon-gamma in mediating the antitumor efficacy of interleukin-12. J Immunother Emphasis Tumor Immunol 17: 71–77

Cesano A, Visonneau S, Clark SC, Santoli D (1993) Cellular and molecular mechanisms of activation of MHC nonrestricted cytotoxic cells by IL-12. J Immunol 151: 2943–2957

Chan SH, Perussia B, Gupta JW, Kobayashi M, Pospisil M, Young HA, Wolf SF, Young D, Clark SC, Trinchieri G (1991) Induction of interferon gamma production by natural killer cell stimulatory factor: characterization of the responder cells and synergy with other inducers. J. Exp Med 173: 869–879

Chehimi J, Starr SE, Frank I, Rengaraju M, Jackson SJ, Llanes C, Kobayashi M, Perussia B, Young D, Nickbarg E et al (1992) Natural killer (NK) cell stimulatory factor increases the cytotoxic activity of NK cells from both healthy donors and human immunodeficiency virus-infected patients. J Exp Med 175: 789–796

Chehimi J, Starr SE, Frank I, D'Andrea A, Ma X, MacGregor RR, Sennelier J, Trinchieri G (1994) Impaired interleukin 12 production in human immunodeficiency virus-infected patients. J Exp Med 179: 1361–1366

Chizzonite R, Truitt T, Desai BB, Nunes P, Podlaski FJ, Stern AS, Gately MK (1992) IL-12-receptor. I. Characterization of the receptor on phytohemagglutinin-activated human lymphoblasts. J Immunol 148: 3117–3124

Chua AO, Chizzonite R, Desai BB, Truitt TP, Nunes P, Minetti LJ, Warrier RR, Presky DH, Levine JF, Gately MK, et al (1994) Expression cloning of a human IL-12 receptor component. A new member of the cytokine receptor superfamily with strong homology to gp130. J Immunol 153: 128–136

Clemons KV, Brummer E, Stevens DA (1994) Cytokine treatment of central nervous system infection: efficacy of interleukin-12 alone and synergy with conventional antifungal therapy in experimental cryptococcosis. Antimicrob Agents Chemother 38: 460–464

Cohen J (1995) IL-12 deaths: explanation and a puzzle [newsl. Science 270: 908

D'Andrea A, Rengaraju M, Valiante NM, Chehimi J, Kubin M, Aste M, Chan SH, Kobayashi M, Young D, Nickbarg E, et al (1992) Production of natural killer cell stimulatory factor (interleukin 12) by peripheral blood mononuclear cells. J Exp Med 176: 1387–1398

D'Andrea A, Aste Amezaga M, Valiante NM, Ma X, Kubin M, Trinchieri G (1993) Interleukin 10 (IL-10) inhibits human lymphocyte interferon gamma-production by suppressing natural killer cell stimulatory factor/IL-12 synthesis in accessory cells. J Exp Med 178: 1041-1048

Desai BB, Quinn PM, Wolitzky AG, Mongini PKA, Chizzonite R, Gately MK (1992) The IL-12 receptor. II. Distribution and regulation of receptor expression. J Immunol 148: 3125–3132

Eng VM, Car BD, Schnyder B, Lorenz M, Lugli S, Aguet M, Anderson TD, Ryffel B, Quesniaux VF (1995) The stimulatory effects of interleukin (IL)-12 on hematopoiesis are antagonized by IL-12-induced interferon gamma in vivo. J Exp Med 181: 1893–1898

Gajewski TF, Renauld JC, Van Pel A, Boon T (1995) Costimulation with B7-1, IL-6, and IL-12 is sufficient for primary generation of murine antitumor cytolytic T lymphocytes in vitro. J Immunol 154:5637-5648
Gately MK (1993) Interleukin-12: a recently discovered cytokine with potential for enhancing cell-mediated immune responses to tumors. Cancer Invest 11:500–506
Gately MK, Desai BB, Wolitzky AG, Quinn PM, Dwyer CM, Podlaski FJ, Familletti PC, Sinigaglia F, Chizzonite R, Gubler U, et al (1991) Regulation of human lymphocyte proliferation by a heterodimeric cytokine, IL-12 (cytotoxic lymphocyte maturation factor). J Immunol 147:874–882
Gavett SH, O'Hearn DJ, Li X, Huang SK, Finkelman FD, Wills Karp M (1995) Interleukin 12 inhibits antigen-induced airway hyperresponsiveness, inflammation, and Th2 cytokine expression in mice. J Exp Med 182:1527–1536
Gazzinelli RT, Wysocka M, Hayashi S, Denkers EY, Hieny S, Caspar P, Trinchieri G, Sher A (1994) Parasite-induced IL-12 stimulates early IFN-gamma synthesis and resistance during acute infection with Toxoplasma gondii. J Immunol 153: 2533–2543
Gearing DP, Cosman D (1991) Homology of the p40 subunit of natural killer cell stimulatory factor (NKSF) with the extracellular domain of the interleukin 6 receptor. Cell 66:9–10
Germann T, Szeliga J, Hess H, Storkel S, Podlaski FJ, Gately MK, Schmitt E, Rude E (1995) Administration of interleukin 12 in combination with type II collagen induces severe arthritis in DBA/1 mice. Proc Natl Acad Sci USA 92:4823–4827
Ghalib HW, Whittle JA, Kubin M, Hashim FA, el Hassan AM, Grabstein KH, Trinchieri G, Reed SG (1995) IL-12 enhances Th1-type responses in human Leishmania donovani infections. J Immunol 154:4623–4629
Gubler U, Chua AO, Schoenhaut DS, Dwyer CM, McComas W, Motyka R, Nabavi N, Wolitzky AG, Quinn PM, Familletti PC et al (1991) Coexpression of two distinct genes is required to generate secreted bioactive cytotoxic lymphocyte maturation factor. Proc Natl Acad Sci USA 88:4143–4147
Heinzel FP, Schoenhaut DS, Rerko RM, Rosser LE, Gately MK (1993) Recombinant interleukin 12 cures mice infected with Leishmania major. J Exp Med 177: 1505–1509
Heinzel FP, Rerko RM, Ling P, Hakimi J, Schoenhaut DS (1994) Interleukin 12 is produced in vivo during endotoxemia and stimulates synthesis of gamma interferon. Infect Immun 62:4244–4249
Heinzel FP, Rerko RM, Ahmed F, Pearlman E (1995) Endogenous IL-12 is required for control of Th2 cytokine responses capable of exacerbating leishmaniasis in normally resistant mice. J Immunol 155:730–739
Hirao A, Takaue Y, Kawano Y, Sato J, Suzue T, Abe T, Saito S, Kawahito M, Okamoto Y, Makimoto A et al (1995) Synergism of interleukin 12, interleukin 3 and serum factor on primitive human hematopoietic progenitor cells. Stem Cells Dayt 13:47–53
Hunter CA, Candolfi E, Subauste C, Van Cleave V, Remington JS (1995) Studies on the role of interleukin-12 in acute murine toxoplasmosis. Immunology 84:16–20
Jacobsen SE, Veiby OP, Smeland EB (1993) Cytotoxic lymphocyte maturation factor (interleukin 12) is a synergistic growth factor for hematopoietic stem cells. J Exp Med 178:413–418
Jacobsen SE, Okkenhaug C, Myklebust J, Veiby OP, Lyman SD (1995) The FLT3 ligand potently and directly stimulates the growth and expansion of primitive murine bone marrow progenitor cells in vitro: synergistic interactions with interleukin (IL) 11, IL-12, and other hematopoietic growth factors. J Exp Med 181:1357–1363

Jacobson NG, Szabo SJ, Weber Nordt RM, Zhong Z, Schreiber RD, Darnell JE Jr, Murphy KM (1995) Interleukin 12 signaling in T helper type 1 (Th1) cells involves tyrosine phosphorylation of signal transducer and activator of transcription (Stat)3 and Stat4. J Exp Med 181:1755–1762

Kobayashi M, Fitz L, Ryan M, Hewick RM, Clark SC, Chan S, Loudon R, Sherman F, Perussia B, Trinchieri G (1989) Identification and purification of natural killer cell stimulatory factor (NKSF), a cytokine with multiple biologic effects on human lymphocytes. J Exp Med 170:827–846

Kobayashi K, Kasama T, Yamazaki J, Hosaka M, Katsura T, Mochizuki T, Soejima K, Nakamura RM (1995) Protection of mice from Mycobacterium avium infection by recombinant interleukin-12. Antimicrob Agents Chemother 39:1369–1371

Kubin M, Chow JM, Trinchieri G (1994a) Differential regulation of interleukin-12 (IL-12), tumor necrosis factor alpha, and IL-1 beta production in human myeloid leukemia cell lines and peripheral blood mononuclear cells. Blood 83:1847–1855

Kubin M, Kamoun M, Trinchieri G (1994b) Interleukin 12 synergizes with B7/CD28 interaction in inducing efficient proliferation and cytokine production of human T cells. J Exp Med 180:211–222

Leder GH, Oppenheim M, Rosenstein M, Lotze MT, Beger HG (1995) Addition of interleukin 12 to low dose interleukin 2 treatment improves antitumor efficacy in vivo. Z Gastroenterol 33:499–502

Macatonia SE, Hosken NA, Litton M, Vieira P, Hsieh CS, Culpepper JA, Wysocka M, Trinchieri G, Murphy KM, O'Garra A (1995) Dendritic cells produce IL-12 and direct the development of Th1 cells from naive CD4+ T cells. J Immunol 154:5071–5079

Maguire HC (1995) Murine recombinant interleukin-12 increases the acquisition of allergic contact dermatitis in the mouse. Int Arch Allergy Immunol 106:166–168

Manetti R, Parronchi P, Giudizi MG, Piccinni MP, Maggi E, Trinchieri G, Romagnani S (1993) Natural killer cell stimulatory factor (interleukin 12 [IL-12]) induces T helper type 1 (Th1)-specific immune responses and inhibits the development of IL-4-producing Th cells. J Exp Med 177:1199–1204

Manetti R, Gerosa F, Giudizi MG, Biagiotti R, Parronchi P, Piccinni MP, Sampognaro S, Maggi E, Romagnani S, Trinchieri G, et al (1994) Interleukin 12 induces stable priming for interferon gamma (IFN-gamma) production during differentiation of human T helper (Th) cells and transient IFN-gamma production in established Th2 cell clones. J Exp Med 179:1273–1283

Mattner F, Fischer S, Guckes S, Jin S, Kaulen H, Schmitt E, Rude E, Germann, T (1993) The interleukin-12 subunit p40 specifically inhibits effects of the interleukin-12 heterodimer. Eur J Immunol 23:2202–2208

Merberg DM, Wolf SF, Clark SC (1992) Sequence similarity between NKSF and the IL-6/G-CSF family (letter). Immunol Today 13:77–78

Metzger DW, Raeder R, Van Cleave VH, Boyle MD (1995) Protection of mice from group A streptococcal skin infection by interleukin-12. J Infect Dis 171:1643–1645

Muller G, Saloga J, Germann T, Bellinghausen I, Mohamadzadeh M, Knop J, Enk AH (1994) Identification and induction of human keratinocyte-derived IL-12. J Clin Inves 94:1799–1805

Muller G, Saloga J, Germann T, Schuler G, Knop J, Enk AH (1995) IL-12 as mediator and adjuvant for the induction of contact sensitivity in vivo. J Immunol 155:4661–4668

Murray HW, Hariprashad J (1995) Interleukin 12 is effective treatment for an established systemic intracellular infection: experimental visceral leishmaniasis. J Exp Med 181:387–391

Nadeau RR, Ostrowski C, Ni Wu G, Liberato DJ (1995) Pharmacokinetics and pharmacodynamics of recombinant human interleukin-12 in male rhesus monkeys. J Pharmacol Exp Ther 274:78–83

Naume B, Johnsen AC, Espevik T, Sundan A (1993) Gene expression and secretion of cytokines and cytokine receptors from highly purified CD56+ natural killer cells stimulated with interleukin-2, interleukin-7 and interleukin-12. Eur J Immunol 23:1831–1838

Neurath MF, Fuss I, Kelsall BL, Stuber E, Strober W (1995) Antibodies to interleukin 12 abrogate established experimental colitis in mice. J Exp Med, 182:1281–1290

Noguchi Y, Richards EC, Chen YT, Old LJ (1995) Influence of interleukin 12 on p53 peptide vaccination against established Meth A sarcoma. Proc Natl Acad Sci USA 92:2219–2223

Orange JS, Wolf SF, Biron CA (1994) Effects of IL-12 on the response and susceptibility to experimental viral infections. J Immunol 152:1253–1264

Orange JS, Salazar Mather TP, Opal SM, Spencer RL, Miller AH, McEwen BS, Biron CA (1995a) Mechanism of interleukin 12-mediated toxicities during experimental viral infections: role of tumor necrosis factor and glucocorticoids. J Exp Med 181: 901–914

Orange JS, Wang B, Terhorst C, Biron CA (1995b) Requirement for natural killer cell-produced interferon gamma in defense against murine cytomegalovirus infection and enhancement of this defense pathway by interleukin 12 administration. J Exp Med 182:1045–1056

Ozmen L, Pericin M, Hakimi J, Chizzonite RA, Wysocka M, Trinchieri G, Gately M, Garotta G (1994) Interleukin 12, interferon gamma, and tumor necrosis factor alpha are the key cytokines of the generalized Shwartzman reaction. J Exp Med 180:907–915

Perussia B, Chan SH, D'Andrea A, Tsuji K, Santoli D, Pospisil M, Young D, Wolf SF, Trinchieri G (1992) Natural killer (NK) cell stimulatory factor or IL-12 has differential effects on the proliferation of TCR-alpha beta+, TCR-gamma delta+ T lymphocytes, and NK cells. J Immunol 149:3495–3502

Podlaski FJ, Nanduri VB, Hulmes JD, Pan YC, Levin W, Danho W, Chizzonite R, Gately MK, Stern AS (1992) Molecular characterization of interleukin 12. Arch Biochem Biophys 294:230–237

Rabinowich H, Herberman RB, Whiteside TL (1993) Differential effects of IL12 and IL2 on expression and function of cellular adhesion molecules on purified human natural killer cells. Cell Immunol 152:481–498

Robertson MJ, Soiffer RJ, Wolf SF, Manley TJ, Donahue C, Young D, Herrmann SH, Ritz J (1992) Response of human natural killer (NK) cells to NK cell stimulatory factor (NKSF): cytolytic activity and proliferation of NK cells are differentially regulated by NKSF. J Exp Med 175:779–788

Salcedo TW, Azzoni L, Wolf SF, Perussia B (1993) Modulation of perforin and granzyme messenger RNA expression in human natural killer cells. J Immunol 151:2511–2520

Saunders BM, Zhan Y, Cheers C (1995) Endogenous interleukin-12 is involved in resistance of mice to Mycobacterium avium complex infection. Infect Immun 63: 4011–4015

Schoenhaut DS, Chua AO, Wolitzky AG, Quinn PM, Dwyer CM, McComas W, Familletti PC, Gately MK, Gubler U (1992) Cloning and expression of murine IL-12. J Immunol 148:3433–3440

Shu U, Kiniwa M, Wu CY, Maliszewski C, Vezzio N, Hakimi J, Gately M, Delespesse G (1995) Activated T cells induce interleukin-12 production by monocytes via CD40-CD40 ligand interaction. Eur J Immunol 25:1125–1128

Sieburth D, Jabs EW, Warrington JA, Li X, Lasota J, LaForgia S, Kelleher K, Huebner K, Wasmuth JJ, Wolf SF (1992) Assignment of genes encoding a unique cytokine (IL12) composed of two unrelated subunits to chromosomes 3 and 5. Genomics 14: 59–62

Stern AS, Podlaski FJ, Hulmes CD, Pan YE, Quinn PM, Wolitzky AG, Familletti PC, Stremlo DL, Truitt T, Chizzonite R, Gately MK (1990) Purification to homogeneity and partial characterization of cytotoxic T lymphocyte maturation factor from human lymphoblastoid cells. Proc Natl Acad Sci USA 87: 6808–6812
Taga T, Kishimoto T (1993) Cytokine receptors and signal transduction. FASEB J 7: 3387–3396
Tare NS, Bowen S, Warrier RR, Carvajal DM, Benjamin WR, Riley JH, Anderson TD, Gately MK (1995) Administration of recombinant interleukin-12 to mice suppresses hematopoiesis in the bone marrow but enhances hematopoiesis in the spleen. J Interferon Cytokine Res 15: 377–383
Trembleau S, Germann T, Gately MK, Adorini L (1995) The role of IL-12 in the induction of organ-specific autoimmune diseases. Immunol Today 16: 383–386
Trinchieri G (1995) Interleukin 12: a proinflammatory cytokine with immunoregulatory functions that bridge innate resistance and antigen-specific adaptive immunity. Annu Rev Immunol 13: 251–276
van der Pouw Kraan TC, Boeije LC, Smeenk RJ, Wijdenes J, Aarden, LA (1995) Prostaglandin-E2 is a potent inhibitor of human interleukin 12 production. J Exp Med 181: 775–779
Vieira LQ, Hondowicz BD, Afonso LC, Wysocka M, Trinchieri G, Scott P (1994) Infection with Leishmania major induces interleukin-12 production in vivo. Immunol Lett 40: 157–161
Voest EE, Kenyon BM, O'Reilly MS, Truitt G, D'Amato RJ, Folkman J (1995) Inhibition of angiogenesis in vivo by interleukin 12. J Natl Cancer Inst 87: 581–586
Wolf SF, Temple PA, Kobayashi M, Young D, Dicig M, Lowe L, Dzialo R, Fitz L, Ferenz C, Hewick RM, et al (1991) Cloning of cDNA for natural killer cell stimulatory factor, a heterodimeric cytokine with multiple biologic effects on T and natural killer cells. J Immunol 146: 307–3081
Wu CY, Demeure C, Kiniwa M, Gately M, Delespesse G (1993) IL-12 induces the production of IFN gamma by neonatal human CD4 T cells. J Immunol 151: 1938–1949
Wysocka M, Kubin M, Vieira LQ, Ozmen L, Garotta G, Scott P, Trinchieri G (1995) Interleukin-12 is required for interferon-gamma production and lethality in lipopolysaccharide-induced shock in mice. Eur J Immunol 25: 672–676
Yang Y, Trinchieri G, Wilson JM (1995) Recombinant IL-12 prevents formation of blocking IgA antibodies to recombinant adenovirus and allows repeated gene therapy to mouse lung. Nat Med 1: 890–893
Zhou P, Sieve MC, Bennett J, Kwon Chung KJ, Tewari RP, Gazzinelli RT, Sher A, Seder RA (1995) IL-12 prevents mortality in mice infected with Histoplasma capsulatum through induction of IFN-gamma. J Immunol 155: 785–795

Peptide Vaccines in Melanoma Patients

A. Knuth and E. Jäger

Introduction

Melanoma is one of the few human tumors of which spontaneous regressions are rarely observed (Balch et al. 1992; Gromet et al. 1978). This observation strongly suggests the presence of antigenic determinants in the tumor that can be recognized by the immune system. Early attempts to activate immunological effectors against metastatic melanoma were based on immunization with irradiated autologous tumor cells. Two patients, SK-29 and MZ-2, with inoperable metastatic melanoma were treated and observed by our group since 1978 and 1982, respectively (Knuth et al. 1984). Both patients received several courses of intradermal immunizations with autologous tumor cells. Both patients experienced a complete regression of all tumor manifestations and up to now have remained free of disease for 19 and 14 years. Based on these favorable clinical developments, extended experimental efforts have been made during the last few years to identify the antigenic determinants involved and to characterize the nature of the suggested immune responses which mediated tumor regression in vivo (Knuth et al. 1991; Knuth et al. 1992).

Cytotoxic T lymphocytes (CTLs) were isolated from melanoma patients, which effectively lyse melanoma cells in vitro (Knuth et al. 1992). Antigenic determinants have been found to be presented by MHC class I and II molecules. The first antigen to be identified, which is recognized by CTLs in a HLA-A1-restricted fashion, was isolated from the melanoma of patient MZ-2 and is designated MAGE-1 (Van der Bruggen et al. 1991). Later, a family of MAGE-1-related genes (MAGE-1, MAGE-3, BAGE, GAGE) was characterized: these genes code for antigens that are expressed in melanomas and some other tumors, but not in normal tissues except testis (Brasseur et al. 1995; Gaugler et al. 1994; Traversari et al. 1992; Van den Eynde et al. 1995; Van der Bruggen et al. 1991).

A second category of antigens derived from differentiation antigens of the melanocyte lineage were found to be recognized by CTLs in melanomas, and are also expressed in normal melanocytes (Bakker et al. 1994; Brichard et al. 1993; Coulie et al. 1994; Kawakami et al. 1994). Several epitopes derived from these self-antigens such as Melan A/MART-1, tyrosinase, gp100/Pmel17, and gp75/TRP-1 have been identified as targets for CTLs and tumor-infiltrating

Symposium in Immunology VI
Eibl/Huber/Peter/Wahn (Eds.)

lymphocytes (TILs) in the context of HLA-A2.1 and other MHC molecules (Kang et al. 1995; Kawakami et al. 1995; Wölfel et al. 1994)

A third group of antigens created by point mutations has been shown to generate strong CTL responses in animal and human tumor systems (Coulie et al. 1995; Mandelboim et al. 1994; Wölfel et al. 1995). Although antigens created by point mutations can be expected to be tumor-specific, it is questionable, to date, whether they appear in a higher frequency in association with certain tumor types and thereby represent useful targets for immunotherapeutic strategies of broader applicability.

Peptides of nine to ten amino acids presented by MHC class I molecules have been identified as the CTL-defined antigenic determinants expressed in tumor and normal tissues. These peptides represent attractive targets for therapeutic immune interventions. Objective tumor regression in single melanoma patients has been observed after adoptive transfer of tumor-infiltrating lymphocyte lines directed against gp100/Pmel17-, tyrosinase-, and gp75-derived epitopes, suggesting that differentiation antigens can serve as tumor rejection antigens (Bakker et al. 1994; Kawakami et al. 1994; Robbins et al. 1994).

Antigenic Peptides as Targets for Spontaneous Cytotoxic T Lymphocyte Reactivity

The spontaneous CTL reactivity against melanoma-associated peptides was determined in melanoma patients and healthy individuals as a basis fo the development of active immunization strategies using antigenic peptides. Up to now, no baseline CTL reactivity against antigens encoded by the MAGE gene family has been found in healthy controls or melanoma patients. In contrast to this, spontaneous CTL reactivity against peptides derived from the differentiation antigens Melan A/MART-1, tyrosinase, and gp100/Pmel17 is frequently detected in melanoma patients and healthy individuals. Remarkably, there is no significant difference in frequency and intensity of CTL responses between melanoma patients and healthy controls (Jäger et al. 1996a; Rivoltini et al. 1995; Visseren et al. 1995).

Induction of Cytotoxic T Lymphocyte Responses with Active Immunization Using Melanoma-Associated Peptides

Preliminary results of phase I trials using antigenic peptides for active immunization are promising. Patients with metastatic melanoma, whose tumors showed an expression of the MAGE genes, Melan A/MART-1, tyrosinase, or gp100/Pmel17, were immunized with the respective antigen-derived peptide with subcutaneous or an intradermal route of immunization. Endpoints of observation were the induction of delayed-type-hypersensitivity reactions (DTH) at the site of peptide inoculation, suggesting peptide-specific local cellular reactions, the induction of peptide-specific CTL after immunization in vivo, and the clinical development of the disease.

Partial responses of metastatic melanoma were reported in three of six patients after three subcutaneous immunizations at monthly intervals with peptides derived from MAGE-3. DTH reactions or effectors mediating tumor regression, however, could not be identified so far (Marchand et al. 1995).

In another study six patients received intradermal injections of melanoma-associated peptides derived from the differentiation antigens Melan A/MART-1 (EAAGIGILTV), tyrosinase (MLLAVLYCL and YMDGTMSQV), and gp100/Pmel17 (YLEPGPVTA and LLDGTATLRL) and the influenza matrix peptide (GILGFVFTL) as a control in a weekly schedule. The signal and internal tyrosinase peptides, and the influenza matrix peptide elicited DTH reactions in five of six patients. No DTH reactions were observed after injection of the Melan A/MART-1- and gp100/Pmel17-derived peptides (Jäger et al. 1996).

Changes of measurable peptide-specific CTL responses against single peptide epitopes after intradermal inoculation of synthetic, melanoma-associated peptides were documented in all patients. Three of six patients developed a CTL response against the Melan A/MART-1-derived peptide, and in two of six patients a CTL response against the signal peptide of tyrosinase (MLLAVLYCL) was observed. One patient showed a decreasing response against the internal peptide of tyrosinase (YMDGTMSQV) after repeated immunizations. A CTL response was not detected against the gp100/Pmel17-derived peptide epitopes prior to or after the vaccination. Baseline reactivity of CTLs directed against the influenza matrix peptide was not altered by peptide inoculation in three of six patients, two of six patients had an increased CTL response, and one of six a decreased CTL response against the influenza matrix peptide after vaccination (Jäger et al 1996). The patterns of CTL responses are listed in Table 1.

Two patients (NW13, NW16) each received a total of three cycles of peptide vaccination within 4 week intervals. In these patients, activation of CTLs induced by the vaccine was maintained under continued peptide injections (Fig. 1a, b).

In two of six patients the initially progressive disease was stabilized. One patient developed facial vitiligo and showed minor regression of lymph node metastasis, possibly resulting from a CTL response to the vaccine (Jäger et al. 1996).

Table 1 Changes in CTL reactivity[a] against different epitopes induced by intradermal peptide injections before vaccination on day 0 (Pre Vac D0) and after the course of vaccination on day 28 (Post Vac D28)

	Melan A								Tyrosinase								gp100/Pmel17								Influenza			
Patient	1 AAGIGILTV				2 EAAGIGILTV				3 MLLAVLYCL				4 YMDGTMSQV				5 YLEPGPVTA				6 LLDGTATLRL				7 GILGFVFTL			
E:T ratio	90	30	10	1	90	30	10	1	90	30	10	1	90	30	10	1	90	30	10	1	90	30	10	1	90	30	10	1
NW 12 Pre Vac D0	2	0	0	0	13	3	0	2					0	0	0	0	0	0	0	0	2	1	0	0	60	43	21	5
NW 12 Post Vac D28	29	19	8	2	13	8	2	4					18	7	4	5	0	0	0	0	0	0	0	0	41	18	11	3
NW 13 Pre Vac D0	14	5	2	0	0	0	0	0	1	1	0	0	0	0	0	0	0	0	0	0	0	1	0	0	19	11	4	3
NW 13 Post Vac D28	22	14	8	2	2	1	1	0	6	3	2	1	3	2	2	0	2	0	0	0	0	0	0	0	41	30	16	4

NW 15	0	0	0	41	17	0	45
	1	0	1	16	7	1	27
	0	0	0	9	2	0	18
Pre Vac D0	0	0	0	3	0	0	3
NW 15	3	0	0	3	0	0	2
	5	1	0	0	0	0	5
	1	0	0	0	0	0	1
Post Vac D28	0	0	0	0	0	0	0
NW 16	57	39	0	1	0	0	21
	34	24	0	0	0	0	17
	18	10	0	0	0	0	13
Pre Vac D0	12	2	0	0	0	0	8
NW 16	48	41	24	2	0	0	63
	19	8	14	6	0	0	55
	8	2	11	1	0	0	48
Post Vac D28	2	4	6	1	0	0	34
NW 28	1	5	0	0	2		11
	5	16	11	8	0		14
	1	3	3	5	2		2
Pre Vac D0	0	0	4	0	1		2
NW 28	21	6	34	10	6		30
	11	25	8	15	7		21
	8	2	1	0	0		12
Post Vac D28	1	1	7	0	4		9

Patient	E:T ratio	Melan A 1 AAGIGILTV	2 EAAGIGILTV	Tyrosinase 3 MLLAVLYCL	4 YMDGTMSQV	gp100/Pmel17 5 YLEPGPVTA	6 LLDGTATLRL	Influenza 7 GILGFVFTL
NW 29 Pre Vac D0	90	9	24	7	14	0		0
	30	12	20	0	8	0		0
	10	14	22	0	5	0		0
	1	2	4	0	1	0		0
NW 29 Post Vac D28	90	10	37	25	21	8		0
	30	8	45	37	0	0		0
	10	1	27	19	0	0		0
	1	0	4	8	0	0		0

[a] Using MLPC assays with peptide-pulsed autologous PBL in vitro, major changes in CTL response were detected for Melan A/MART-1 (NW12, NW13, NW28, NW29), the signal peptide of tyrosinase (NW16, NW28, NW29), the internal peptide of tyrosinase (NW15), and the influenza matrix peptide (NW13, NW15, NW16, NW28) epitopes. Specific target lysis was tested at epitope:CTL (E:T) ratios of 1, 10, 30, 90:1.

[b] The patients are designated NW12, NW13, NW15, NW16, NW28, and NW29.

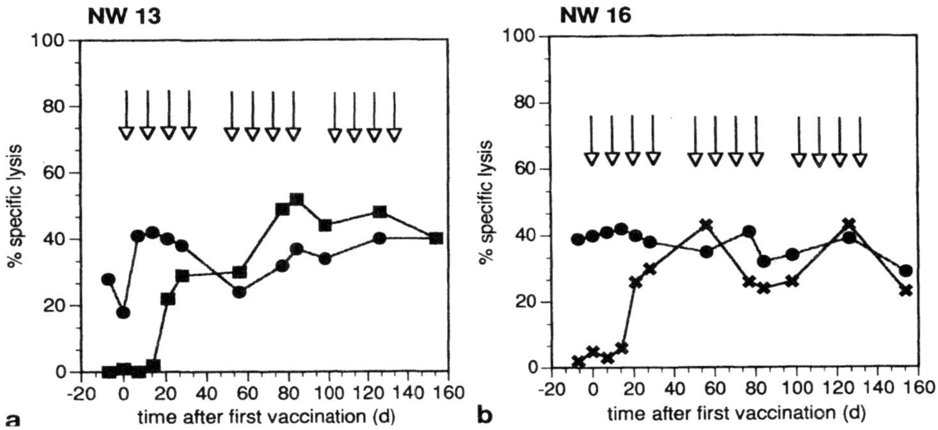

Fig. 1a,b. Induction of peptide-specific CTLs by intradermal immunization with the natural Melan A/MART-1 nonamer peptide epitope in patient NW13 (**a**) and with the signal peptide of tyrosinase in patient NW16 (**b**). A significant increase in the specific CTL response against T2 cells pulsed with the Melan A/MART-1 derived nonamer (**a**) and the tyrosinase peptide (**b**) was maintained during repeated vaccinations within 4-week intervals (*arrows* indicate the days of vaccination)

Immunoselection In Vivo after Immunization with Melanoma-Associated Peptides

Three patients, who had received repeated injections of melanoma associated peptides derived from Melan A/MART-1, tyrosinase, and gp100/Pmel17 showed an increased CTL response against the Melan A/MART-1- and the tyrosinase-derived signal peptide which was maintained under continued immunization. One patient showed regression of Melan A/MART-1-positive axillary lymph node metastasis in the presence of CTL reactivity against Melan A/MART-1. Subsequently, local tumor growth and new metastatic lesions in the lung, liver, and spleen were diagnosed. Biopsies from the local recurrence and various metastatic sites showed a complete loss of Melan A/MART-1 expression.

The second patient had two metastatic sites in the left leg, one of which was positive for tyrosinase. With continued immunization, the tyrosinase-positive lesion completely regressed in the presence of CTLs directed against the signal peptide of tyrosinase, whereas the other lesion continuously increased (Jäger et al. 1996).

The third patient presented with local recurrence in the left supraclavicular region. The lesion was resected and the tumor tissue was found to express Melan A/MART-1 and tyrosinase. The patient received repeated injections of Melan A/MART-1- and tyrosinase-derived peptides and weak, peptide-specific CTL responses directed against the Melan A/MART-1 and the signal peptide of tyrosinase were detected. Subsequently, the patient was again diagnosed with a local recurrence; the incompletely resected tumor tissue showed a less intense expression of Melan A/MART-1 and tyrosinase. Vaccination was continued with the Melan A/MART-1- and tyrosinase-derived peptides including granulocyte-macrophage colony-stimulating factor (GM-CSF) as an adjuvant. CTL responses against Melan A/MART-1 and the signal peptide of tyrosinase were enhanced after GM-CSF administration. Initially, local tumorous infiltrates in the skin completely regressed in the presence of a strong Melan A/MART-1- and tyrosinase CTL reactivity. Then, local tumor growth was observed; the resected tumor tissue was negative for Melan A/MART-1- and tyrosinase expression (Jäger, unpublished data).

These observations strongly suggest that regression of melanomas expressing melanoma-associated differentiation antigens is mediated by antigen-specific CTLs. The presence of antigen-specific CTLs, however, may also support the selection of antigen-loss variants.

Enhancement of Immune Responses to Melanoma-Associated Peptides with Systemic Granulocyte-Macrophage Colony-Stimulating Factor

Peptides alone, injected intradermally, elicit cellular immune responses in vivo. Antigen constitution may be enhanced after intradermal peptide injection by an increased frequency of antigen-presenting cells (APCs). Dermal APCs such as dendritic Langerhans' cells are stimulated by GM-CSF (Caux et al. 1992). The effect of systemic GM-CSF as an adjuvant on immune responses to melanoma-associated peptides in vivo was evaluated by monitoring the generation of DTH reactions, the immunohistochemical characterization of DTH-constituting elements and the assessment of peptide-specific CTL responses. Enhanced DTH reactions and CD8+ CTL responses were observed after treatment with systemic GM-CSF. Immunohistochemical characterization of DTH-constituting elements revealed infiltrates of CD4+ and CD8+ T lymphocytes and a strong expression of interleukin-2 (IL-2) and interferon-γ, suggesting the activation of CD4+ T helper type 1 cells (Th1) and CD8+ CTLs by peptides presented by MHC class I molecules of dermal APC. Objective tumor regression was documented in all patients vaccinated (three of three). It is concluded that systemic GM-CSF enhances immune responses to melanoma-associated peptides and supports CTL-mediated tumor rejection in vivo (Jäger et al. 1996)

Future Perspectives

Future perspectives of tumor vaccine development are focused on more potent strategies of immunization. Vaccination with whole proteins containing multiple, relevant antigenic epitopes may increase the chance of multidirectional B- and T-cell activation. Adjuvants may enhance the immunogenicity of peptides and proteins by activating costimulatory factors and mediating the production of cytokines (Matzinger 1994). Autologous dendritic cells pulsed with peptides or proteins in vitro, or transfected with the relevant genes, may effectively activate both class-I- and class-II-restricted T lymphocytes in vivo (Alijagic et al. 1995; Schirmbeck et al. 1995). Cytokines have been found to play a key role in T-cell activation. GM-CSF has been shown to induce long-lasting Th1 and CD8+ T cell responses by efficient activation of dendritic cells in vivo (Dranoff et al. 1993). IL-12 is a potent activator of Th1 and CD8+ T lymphocytes. At low doses it has been shown to mediate complete tumor regression when used as an adjuvant to immunization with a mutant peptide of p53 in an animal model (Noguchi et al. 1995). The identification of other tumor antigens will give a broader basis for multidirectional immunization strategies to prevent tumor escape by immunoselection of antigen-loss variants (Jäger et al. 1996).

References

Alijagic S, Müller P, Artuc M, Jurgovsky K, Czarnetzki BM, Schadendorf D (1995) Dendritic cells generated from peripheral blood transfected with human tyrosinase induce specific T cell activation. Eur J Immunol 25:3100–3107

Bakker AB, Schreurs MWJ, deBoer AJ, Kawakami Y, Rosenberg SA, Adema GJ, Figdor CG (1994) Melanocyte lineage-specific antigen gp100 is recognized by melanoma-derived tumor-infiltrating lymphocytes. J Exp Med, 179:1005–1009

Balch CM, Houghton AN, Milton GW, Soong SJ (1992) Cutaneous Melanoma. Lippincott, Philadelphia

Brasseur F, Rimoldi D, Lienard D, Lethe B, Carrel S, Arienti F, Suter L, Vanwijck R, Bourlond A, Humblet Y, Vacca A, Conese M, Lahaye T, Degiovanni G, Deraemaecker R, Beauduin M, Sastre X, Salamon E, Dreno B., Knuth A, Jäger E, Chevreau C, Suciu S, Lachapelle J-M, Pouillart P, Parmiani G, Lejeune F, Cerottini J-C, Boon T, Marchand M (1995) Expression of MAGE genes in primary and metastatic cutaneous melanoma. Int J Cancer 63:375–380

Brichard V, Van Pel A, Wölfel T, Wölfel C, DePlaen E, Lethe B, Coulie P, Boon T (1993) The tyrosinase gene codes for an antigen recognized by autologous cytolytic T lymphocytes on HLA-A2 melanomas. J Exp Med 178:489–495

Caux C, Dezutter-Dambuyant C, Schmitt D (1992) GM-CSF and TNF-α cooperate in the generation of dendritic Langerhans cells. Nature 360:258-261

Coulie PG, Brichard V, Van Pel A, Wölfel T, Schneider J, Traversari C, Mattei S, DePlaen E, Lurquin C, Szikora J-P, Renauld J-C, Boon T (1994) A new gene coding for a differentiation antigen recognized by autologous cytolytic T lymphocytes on HLA-A2 melanomas. J Exp Med 180:35–42

Coulie PG, Lehmann F, Lethe B, Hermann J, Lurquin C, Andrawiss M, Boon T (1995) A mutated intron sequence codes for an antigenic peptide recognized by cytolytic T lymphocytes on a human melanoma. Proc Natl Acad Sci USA 92:7976–7980

Dranoff G, Jaffee E, Lazenbry A, Golumbek P, Levitsky H, Brose K, Jeckson V, Hamada H, Pardoll D, Mulligan R (1993) Vaccination with irradiated tumor cells engineered to secrete murine granulocyte-macrophage colony-stimulating factor stimulates potent, specific, and long-lasting anti-tumor immunity. Proc Natl Acad Sci USA 90:3539–3543

Gaugler B, Van den Eynde B, van der Bruggen P, Romero P, Gaforio JJ, DePlaen E, Lethe B, Brasseur F, Boon T (1994) Human gene MAGE-3 codes for an antigen recognized on a melanoma by autologous cytolytic T lymphocytes. J Exp Med 179:921–930

Gromet MA, Epstein WL, Blois MS (1978) The regressing thin malignant melanoma: a distinctive lesion with metastatic potential. Cancer 42:2282–2292

Jäger E, Bernhard H, Romero P, Ringhoffer M, Arand M, Karbach J, Ilsemann C, Hagedorn M, Knuth A (1996a) Generation of cytotoxic T cell responses with synthetic melanoma associated peptides in vivo: implications for tumor vaccines with melanoma associated antigens. Int J Cancer (In Press)

Jäger E, Ringhoffer M, Dienes H-P, Arand M, Karbach J, Jäger D, Ilsemann C, Hagedorn M, Oesch F, Knuth A (1996b) Granulocyte macrophage colony-stimulating factor enhances immune responses to melanoma associated peptides in vivo. Int J Cancer (In press)

Jäger E, Ringhoffer M, Karbach J, Arand M, Oesch F, Knuth A (1996c) Inverse relationship of melanocyte differentiation antigen expression in melanoma: evidence for immunoselection of antigen-loss variants in vivo. Int J Cances (In press)

Kang XQ, Kawakami Y, El-Gamil M, Wang R, Sakaguchi K, Yannelli JR, Appella E, Rosenberg SA (1995) Identification of a tyrosinase epitope recognized by HLA-A24-restricted, tumor-infiltrating lymphocytes. J Immunol 155:1343–1348

Kawakami Y, Eliyahu S, Delgado CH, Robins PF, Rivoltini L, Topalian SL, Miki T, Rosenberg SA (1994a) Cloning of the gene coding for a shared human melanoma antigen recognized by autologous T cells infiltrating into tumor. Proc Natl Acad Sci USA 91:3525–35191

Kawakami Y, Eliyahu S, Delgado CH, Robbins PF, Sakaguchi K, Appella E, Yannelli JR, Adema GJ, Miki T, Rosenberg SA (1994b) Identification of a human melanoma antigen recognized by tumor-infiltrating lymphocytes associated with in vivo tumor rejection. Proc Natl Acad Sci USA 91:6458–6462

Kawakami Y, Eliyahu S, Jennings C, Sakaguchi K, Kang XQ, Southwood S, Robbins PF, Sette A, Appella E, Rosenberg SA (1995) Recognition of multiple epitopes in the human melanoma antigen gp100 by tumor-infiltrating lymphocytes associated with in vivo tumor regression. J Immunol 154:3961–3968

Knuth A, Danowski B, Oettgen HF, Old LJ (1984) T-cell-mediated cytotoxicity against autologous malignant melanoma: analysis with interleukin-2-dependent T-cell cultures. Proc Natl Acad Sci USA 81:3511–3515

Knuth A, Wölfel T, Meyer zum Büschenfelde K-H (1991) Cellular and humoral responses against cancer: implications for cancer vaccines. Curr Opin Immunol 3:659–664

Knuth A, Wölfel T, Meyer zum Büschenfelde K-H (1992) T cell responses to human malignant tumours. Cancer Surv 13:39–52

Mandelboim O, Berke G, Fridkin M, Feldman M, Eisenstein M, Eisenbach L (1994) CTL induction by a tumour-associated antigen octapeptide derived from a murine lung carcinoma. Nature 369:67–71

Marchand M, Weymants P, Rankin E, Arienti F, Belli F, Parmiani G, Cascinelli N, Bourlond A, Vanwjick R, Humblet Y, Canon J-L, Laurent C, Naeyaert J-M, Plagne R, Deraemaeker R, Knuth A, Jäger E, Brasseur F, Herman J, Coulie PG, Boon T (1995) Tumor regression responses in melanoma patients treated with a peptide encoded by gene MAGE-3. Int J Cancer 63:883–885

Matzinger P (1994) Tolerance, danger, and the extended family. Annu Rev Immunol 12:991–1045

Noguchi Y, Richards EC, Chen YT, Old LJ (1995) Influence of interleukin-12 on p53 peptide vaccination against established Meth A sarcoma. Proc Natl Acad Sci USA 92:2219–2223

Rivoltini L, Kawakami Y, Sakaguchi K, Southwood S, Sette A, Robbins PF, Marincola FM, Salgaller ML, Yannelli JR, Appella E, Rosenberg SA (1995) Induction of tumor-reactive CTL from peripheral blood and tumor-infiltrating lymphocytes of melanoma patients by in vitro stimulation with an immunodominant peptide of the human melanoma antigen MART-1. J Immunol 154:2257-2265

Robbins PF, El-Gamil M, Kawakami Y, Rosenberg SA (1994) Recognition of tyrosinase by tumor-infiltrating lymphocytes from a patient responding to immunotherapy. Cancer Res 54:3124–3126

Schirmbeck R, Melber K, Reimann J (1995) Hepatitis B virus small surface antigen particles are processed in a novel endosomal pathway for major histocompatibility complex class I-restricted epitope presentation. Eur J Immunol 25:1063-1070

Traversari C, van der Bruggen P, Luescher IF, Lurquin C, Chomez P, van Pel A, DePlaen E, Amarcostesec A, Boon T (1992) A nonapeptide encoded by human gene MAGE-1 is recognized on HLA-A1 by cytolytic T-lymphocytes directed against tumor antigen MZ2-E. J Exp Med 176:1453–1457

Van den Eynde B, Peeters O, De Backer O, Gaugler B, Lucas S, Boon T (1995) A new family of genes coding for an antigen recognized by autologous cytolytic T lymphocytes on a human melanoma. J Exp Med 182:689–698

Van der Bruggen P, Traversari C, Chomez P, Lurquin C, De Plaen E, Van den Eynde B, Knuth A, Boon T (1991) A gene encoding an antigen recognized by cytolytic T lymphocytes on a human melanoma. Science 254:1643–1647

Visseren MJW, van Elsas A, van der Voort EIH, Ressing ME, Kast WM, Schrier PI, Melief CJM (1995) CTL specific for the tyrosinase autoantigen can be induced from healthy donor blood to lyse melanoma cells. J Immunol 154:3991–3998

Wölfel T, Hauer M, Schneider J, Serrano M, Wölfel C, Klehmann-Hieb E, DePlaen E, Hankeln T, Meyer zum Büschenfelde K-H, Beach D (1995) A p16INK4a-insensitive CDK4 mutant targeted by cytolytic T lymphocytes in a human melanoma. Science 269:1281–1284

Wölfel T, Schneider J, Meyer zum Büschenfelde K-H, Rammensee H-G, Rötzschke O, Falk K (1994) Isolation of naturally processed peptides recognized by cytolytic T lymphocytes (CTL) on human melanoma cells in association with HLA-A2.1. Int J Cancer 57:413–418

Ras Peptide Vaccines

G. GAUDERNACK

Introduction

Molecularly defined cancer vaccines have become a clinical realityas more and more tumor antigens are being characterized. One of the first cancer vaccine clinical studies was a pilot phase I/II trial of a ras oncopeptide vaccine, involving five patients with inoperable pancreatic cancer [1, 2].The ras peptide vaccine is targeted against mutations in the ras family of oncogenes (reviewed in [3]), a form of genetic lesion found in 20%–30% of all human cancers. The ras peptide vaccine is primarily designed to stimulate CD4+helper T (Th) cells. In particular, the CD4+ helper Th1 cell subset has been recognized for its importance in initiating and controlling protective cellular immune responses, and may act either directly on the tumor cells or indirectly by triggering an effector cascade of cytotoxic T cells (CTLs), natural killer cells, and activated macrophages. The experiments with human cell cultures providing evidence for the immunogenicity of mutant p21 ras and its peptides, as well as studies in animal models form the platform for the ras peptide vaccines now being tested in clinical protocols.

Ras Proto-oncogene Mutations in Human Cancer

The mechanism leading to cancer involves mutations which result in multiple changes in the genome of the cancer cell. The majority of these genetic changes that have been characterized affect pivotal regulatory molecules involved in the control of cell division and cell death. These key genetic alterations are obvious targets for various forms of specific tumor therapy.

Point mutations have been found in a number of oncogenes and tumor suppressor genes, and in human cancer the first oncogene described which has a point mutation was a member of the ras gene family (for a review see [3]). We have focused on the ras oncogenes as candidate targets for immunotherapy for several reasons. Firstly, the number of different ras mutations that are found in human malignancies is limited, and these mutations are confined to three positions (12, 13, and 61) of the ras protein. Secondly, oncogenic ras mutations are found in about one-third of all human cancers

Symposium in Immunology VI
Eibl/Huber/Peter/Wahn (Eds.)

(reviewed in[3]); in particular, such mutations are frequently found in pancreatic carcinomas (90%–95%), colorectal carcinomas (40%–50%); and lung adenocarcinomas (50%). Thirdly mutations in ras oncogenes can easily be detected in cancer biopsies and in biopsies from premalignant lesions by highly sensitive PCR-based techniques. Finally, although mutant p21 ras proteins are mainly found in the cytoplasm, they can also be detected in extracellular body fluids such as urine [4, 5] in cancer patients. Mutant p21 ras may therefore be expected to trigger immune responses in the CD4+ helper subset of T cells following exogenous uptake of p21 ras by antigen presenting cells (APCs), as well as CD8+ CTL responses.

Since the spectrum of ras mutations occurring in human cancer is so limited, relatively few synthetic peptides will be sufficient to prepare vaccines for the majority of patients having a cancer with a ras mutation. Considering the fact that cancer is a very complex disease, an oncopeptide vaccine based on mutant ras peptides would therefore seem to get as close to a "general" cancer vaccine as one could hope for.

T-Cell Immunosurveillance of Cancer

The lack of defined peptide targets for antitumor immunity has long hampered the development of a specific immunotherapy of cancer based on vaccination. Identification of potentially immunogenic peptides resulting from genetic alterations within cancer cells and characterization of the various components in the immune response against such peptides has therefore become a central area of research in cancer immunology.

T cells may act as a form of quality control of the genome, and this is the basis for immunosurveillance against cancer. Recently, evidence for this mechanism has come from the demonstration of two newly described tumor rejection antigens in human melanomas that were found to be encoded by mutations unique to the melanoma cells [6, 7].

Paradoxically, cancer develops in patients with a functional immune system. This indicates that T cell surveillance may never get started in most cancer patients. The reason for this is that the most cancer cells lack important costimulatory molecules required for the initiation of a T-cell response [8]. To overcome this problem, two complementary approaches have been designed. In one approach, tumor cells are converted to APCs by gene transfection [8]. In the other approach, professional APCs are "dressed up" like cancer cells by loading them with a tumor-specific antigen, such as a ras peptide [1]. This can be done either ex vivo or in vivo and represents the basic principle behind a molecularly defined cancer vaccine.

T-Cell Responses against Mutant p21 Ras and Ras-Derived Peptides

In order to provide an experimental basis for development of cancer vaccines and immunotherapy targeted against mutations in the ras oncogenes, we and others have tested the capacity of synthetic ras peptides to elicit mutation-specific T-cell responses. Jung and Schluesner [8], and subsequently a number of reports from our laboratory [10–17] demonstrated that mutation-specific T-cell responses could be induced in vitro in man. Similar findings were made in mice immunized with synthetic ras peptides in vivo [18].

In normal human donor T cells, responses specific for individual ras mutations can be elicited by in vitro stimulation with synthetic ras peptides [8–17, 19]. Delectable T-cell responses only appear after repeated peptide stimulation over a period of several weeks [9, 10, 13, 19]. Cell lines resulting from these in vitro stimulations have been reported to be specific for the particular mutation represented by the immunizing peptide [9, 19]. The cloning of responding T cells [10, 12, 13] has allowed a more detailed characterization of the basic requirements for T-cell recognition of mutant ras peptides. As observed with T-cell lines, most T-cell clones confirm the exquisite specificity for the single amino acid substitution resulting from the mutation. In some instances, however, cross-reactivity with other mutant ras peptides as well as with the wild-type peptide has been observed [12]. Such broadly reactive T-cell clones have not been a frequent observation, and the phenomenon may be related to the presence of a T-cell receptor with a particularly high affinity.

T-cell responses were obtained against peptides encompassing both mutational hotspots at position 12 and 13 of p21 ras. Attempts to generate T-cell responses against peptides encompassing the mutational hotspot at position 61 by in vitro stimulation of T cells from normal human donors have been less successful. This may be related to a more restricted binding to HLA molecules by such peptides, analogous to that described in mice, where only some amino acid substitutions at position 61 may allow the formation of a class II aggretope [19]. A crucial finding was that ras peptide binding to HLA class II molecules is promiscuous, involving all three class II isotypes [13]. The length of the peptides used and their relative position in p21 ras indicates that many different peptides are immunogenic and are capable of binding to HLA-class II molecules [9, 10, 12, 13, 19]. We have used panels of peptides of different lengths and T-cell clones restricted by various HLA molecules in order to define core binding sequences and consensus peptide sequences capable of binding a large number of HLA class II molecules for use in vaccination protocols [12, 13, 21].

Following the observation that mutant ras peptides can give rise to T-cell responses in normal individuals, we investigated T-cell responses against mutant ras in cancer patients [11, 15]. In these studies, attempts were made to detect spontaneous ("recall") T-cell responses in patients carrying tumors where ras mutations commonly occur. These studies were done without prior determination of an actual ras mutation in the patients. It turned out that recall type T-cell responses against single ras mutations could occasionally be detected, and we detected such T-cell responses in patients with follicular thyroid carcinomas [11] and colorectal carcinomas [15].

Gedde-Dahl et al. [11], using paramagnetic particles coated with a monoclonal antibody against CD45RO, demonstrated that T cells specific for a 61 Gln→Leu mutation belonged to the memory T-cell population. This finding strongly argued in favor of a previous exposure of these T cells to a corresponding peptide in this cancer patient. In a recent report by Quin el al. [22], a high proportion of patients with pancreatic carcinomas were able to respond to a peptide having the common 12 Gly→Asp substitution. In some of these cases, the responding T cells were cloned and studied in detail [11,15]. The T-cell clones generated from the peripheral blood of these patients always displayed the same high degree of specificity for a single mutation as seen in the primary responses of the patients.

When tumor material from the responding patients was tested for the presence of the corresponding ras mutation, it could in no case be detected [11, 15]. One explanation for this puzzling observation is that in the rare cases where a T-cell response is generated against the ras mutation of a tumor, cells harboring the mutation may be eliminated, and cancer clones lacking the mutation may selectively survive.

Processing of p21 Ras Protein in Professional Antigen Presenting Cells and Tumor Cells

The synthetic peptides initially used for immunizing mice or stimulating human T cells in culture were designed mainly on the basis of guesswork. They were made to encompass the relevant amino acid substitution in order to ensure specificity for a particular mutation, and they were long enough to allow some degree of intracellular processing/trimming. Once it was established that these peptides were immunogenic, it became an issue of great importance to confirm that T cells generated by stimulation with synthetic mutant ras peptides could also recognize corresponding epitopes derived from the p21 ras protein by natural processing.

Mutant p21 proteins can be detected extracellularly in cancer patients [4, 5]. An antiras immune response may therefore be initiated through uptake and subsequent presentation by professional APCs. Many studies to adress this important question have been performed, mainly in mouse model systems. Peace et al. [18] have shown that ras-mutation-specific T-cell lines generated after immunization of mice with synthetic peptides can also be stimulated by the corresponding mutant p21 following processing in APCs.

These authors demonstrated that mutant p21 is also immunogenic in vivo [23]. In this reverse experiment, the Th cells generated were able to recognize synthetic peptides carrying the same mutation. Similar results were observed by others who immunized mice with either synthetic peptides carrying mutations at position 12 (12 gly→Val; [24]) or recombinant p21 ras (12 Gly→Arg; [25]. In the latter case, the immunized mice were protected against a subsequent challenge with tumor cells carrying the same mutation, but it is not clear if this immune response involved CD4+ T cells. In humans, both T-cell clones derived from cancer patients [11, 17] and peripheral blood T cells from cancer patients [22] can recognize mutant p21 ras following processing and presentation by professional APCs. In summary, these experiments provide evidence for processing of p21 ras to yield partly overlapping epitopes encompassing the mutational hotspot at position 61 [16] and epitopes including the mutational hotspot at position 12 [22].

Exogenous processing is probably essential for the initiation of an immune response against mutant ras in cancer patients, since most cancer cells lack essential accessory molecules and therefore may anergize rather than stimulate T cells with receptors for tumor specific peptide/MHC complexes. Once an immune response against a cancer-specific peptide has been initiated this response may either indirectly or directly influence the growth of the tumor. For the direct recognition of mutant ras peptides presented by MHC molecules on cancer cells, p21 ras has to be processed in the cancer cell to yield relevant peptide fragments for binding to MHC class I or class II molecules.

A number of experiments in mouse model systems have addressed the important question of endogenous processing of p21 ras in target cells. Following immunization of mice with recombinant vaccinia constructs expressing mutant or normal ras, CD8+ CTL lines were isolated. These cell lines were able to kill vaccinia-virus-infected target cells, demonstrating that endogenous processing to yield a peptide fragment(s) capable of binding to MHC class I molecules had taken place [26]. Two epitopes corresponding to known murine class I binding motifs were identified (amino acid 60–67, encompassing the mutation at position 61, and 152–159 representing a native part of the sequence). These CTLs were also able to kill target cells incubated with both of these peptides, but evidently did not kill target cells expressing low level of wild-type p21. Direct evidence for endogenous processing of mutant p21 ras was also provided by experiments showing that 61 Gln→Leu-specific CD8+ CTL, generated by in vitro priming, could lyse fibroblasts transfected with a ras gene carrying this mutation [27]. Recently, similar findings were reported for a 12 Gly→Val mutation [28].

In the human system evidence exists for endogenous processing which results in peptides that bind to HLA class II and class I molecules. Direct evidence for involvement of the class II processing pathway was provided by Chicz et al. using a biochemical approach [29]. They identified a p21 ras-derived peptide in an acid eluate from DR8 molecules purified from an Epstein-

Barr virus (EBV)-transformed B-cell line. Recently, Tsang et al. [19] generated 12 Gly→Val-specific CD4+T-cell lines from normal donors and colorectal cancer patients by in vitro peptide stimulation. Some of these cell lines were subsequently shown to be able to lyse EBV blasts transfected with a mutated ras gene, but not with a normal ras gene [19]. These results confirm the biochemical finding that ras, which is a cytoplasmic protein, can be processed for the class II pathway, and demonstrate that processing also yields an epitope which includes position 12. Fossum et al. [30] provided indirect evidence for the processing of p21 ras with a 13 Gly→Asp mutation in the HCT 116 colorectal cancer cell line carrying this mutation. HCT116 cells were killed by CD8+ CTLs generated from a colorectal cancer patient who responded to this mutation [15]. In this case, HLA-B44 was identified as the peptide-presenting molecule, but the peptide epitope could not be identified. In another approach, a ras peptide encompassing the 61 Gln→Leu mutation and carrying a HLA-A2 binding motif was used to generate CD8+ CTLs in vitro [31]. These CTLs lysed the target cells which were pulsed with the peptide but were unable to kill transfectants carrying this mutation. The lack of evidence for processing in this case may be due to a low affinity T-cell receptor carried by these CTLs, since the in vitro method for T-cell stimulation used in these experiments allows selection of low affinity precursor T cells from the repertoire of nonimmunized donors.

Presentation and Binding of Ras Peptides to HLA Molecules

In the search for synthetic ras peptides for the purpose of vaccination, it is important that the candidate peptide vaccine is capable of eliciting an immune response in the majority of the individuals vaccinated. For a single peptide this may not be achieved, since most peptides will only bind to certain HLA molecules due to the stringent structural requirement for such binding (review in [32]).

HLA-Class II Promiscuity in Ras Peptide Binding

While class I peptide binding motifs are well defined and to some degree can be predicted from the pocket structure of the MHC molecules, the interaction sites or anchors in class II binding peptides are more degenerate in their specificity [32]. This forms the basis for the promiscuous binding of some peptides to many HLA class II molecules. A large number of experiments have now demonstrated that this is the case for ras peptides. Mutant ras peptides bind to the gene products of many alleles within the HLA-DQ and -DR loci [9–17, 19, 21] and were also one of the first peptides which were found to be recognized in the context of an HLA-DP molecule [13]. The promiscuous nature of ras peptide binding to HLA-class II molecules allows the assumption that every individual will have one or more types of class II molecules that can present a given ras peptide. Cancer patients can therefore be given a ras peptide vaccine without prior selection based on the presence of a certain type of HLA molecule. This greatly facilitates the recruitment of patients for entry into ras peptide vaccine protocols.

HLA-Class I and Peptide Motifs

Little is known about the binding of ras peptides to HLA class I molecules. Biochemical binding studies have shown binding of a 61 Gln→Leu peptide carrying a typical binding motif to HLA-A2 [31], and this peptide could also generate CD8+ CTLs after in vitro stimulation. The peptide encompassing a 12 Gly→Asp mutation and presented by HLA-B44 (see above) remains to be characterized. Peptide binding to HLA class I molecules is, however, a rapidly expanding field, and the list of new HLA-class I binding motifs is growing every month. One rational approach to the development of peptide vaccines is to search for class I motifs that match the class I molecules present in cancer patients in whom a ras mutation has been detected. Synthetic peptides containing the relevant mutation and binding motif can then be tested in order to tailor an individual vaccine for that patient. This is an attractive possibility, since combinations of peptide vaccines representing overlapping epitopes for Th cells and $CD8^+$ CTLs may allow a concerted activation of the two subsets for a coordinated and more efficient response. Studies to test this possibility are ongoing in our laboratory.

Immunization Protocols and Vaccine Trials

Much has already been achieved with respect to defining candidate ras peptide vaccines. Data from our pilot phaseI/II study on patients with inoperable pancreas cancer indicate that even in patients with terminal cancer, a ras-mutation-specific response may be initiated by several rounds of vaccination. These patients showed no sign of ras-specific immunity before the start of vaccination, and no side effects caused by the vaccine were observed [1, 2].

One important observation made in this study was the transient nature of the T-cell response as measured in peripheral blood samples obtained after vaccination [1, 2]. It is conceivable that this will also be observed with other vaccine protocols involving patients with a large tumor mass. Methods for obtaining T cells from the tumor site for functional studies are therefore required. In a recent melanoma vaccine study, evidence was obtained for the presence of peptide-specific T cells both at the site of injection and at a distant metastasis, while no reactivity could detected in peripheral blood [33]. In our new ras vaccine protocols we have tried to get around this by choosing patients where the bulk of the tumor has been removed by surgery. We thus vaccinate pancreatic carcinoma patients following radical operation (Whipple operated) and colorectal cancer patients in dukes stages B and C following primary surgery. These patients have minimal residual disease and hopefully, vaccination may give rise to T-cell responses that can be followed over time. We can follow the presence of bone marrow and blood micrometastasis in these patients and correlate T-cell responses with the fate of micrometastatic cancer cells. These observations may give early information on tumor response.

Fine tuning of the vaccination protocol in various groups of patients will be necessary. In particular, more research is needed in order to define, purify, and possibly also recruit by the use of suitable cytokines, optimal APCs. This approach is presently much in focus and there is already some evidence for in vivo efficacy [33]. Direct injection of peptides as such or of peptide conjugates tailored to initiate strong immune responses of the desired type will also have high priority.

Emphasis so far has been on therapeutic vaccines, and all clinical protocols to date are of this type. For some cancers, where patients at risk can be identified by genetic testing, it may also be considered to give the vaccine prophylactically. This is particularly relevant when a genetic lesion can be predicted to occur with great probability. Before this can be tested in healthy donors, the effect of preexisting immunity on the important early phase of cancer development must be studied in animal model systems.

References

1. Gjertsen MK, Bakka A, Breivik J, Sæterdal I, Solheim BG, Søreide O, Thorsby E, Gaudernack G (1995) Vaccination with mutant ras peptides and induction of T-cell responsiveness in pancreatic carcinoma patients carrying the corresponding *RAS* mutation. The Lancet 346:1399–1400
2. Gjertsen MK, Bakka A, Breivik J, Sæterdal I, Gedde-Dahl III T, Stokke KT, Solheim B, Egge TS, Søreide O, Thorsby E, Gaudernack G (1996) Ex vivo ras peptide vaccination in patients with advanced pancreatic cancer: results of a phaseI/II study. Int J Cancer 65:450–453
3. Bos JL (1989) Ras oncogenes in human cancer: a review. Cancer Res 49: 4682–4689
4. Niman H, Thompson A, Yu A, Markman M, Willems J, Herwig H, Habib N, Wood C, Houghten R, Lerner R (1985) Anti-peptide antibodies detect oncogene-related proteins in urine. Proc Natl Acad Sci USA 82:7924–7928
5. Brandt-Rauf PW (1991) Oncogen proteins as biomarkers in the molecular epidemiology of occupational carcinogenesis. Int Arch Occup Environ Health 63:1–8

6. Coulie PG, Lehmann F, Lethé B, Lurquin C, Adrawiss M, Boon T (1995) A mutated intron sequence codes for an antigenic peptide recognized by cytolytic T lymphocytes on a human melanoma. Proc Natl Acad Sci USA 92: 7976–7980
7. Wölfel T, Hauer M, Schneider J, Serrano M, Wölfel C, Kleinmann-Hieb E, De Plaen E, Hankeln T, Meyer zum Büschenfelde K-H, Beach D (1995) A p16^{INK4a}-insensitive CDK4 mutant targeted by cytolytic T lymphocytes in a human melanoma. Science 269:1281–1284
8. Chen L, Ashe S, Brady WA, Hellström I, Hellström KE, McGowan P, Lindsey PS (1992) Costimulation of antitumor immunity by the B7 counterreceptor for the T lymphocyte molecules CD28 andCTLA-4. Cell 71:1093–1102
9. Jung S, Schluesner HJ (1991) Human T lymphocytes recognize a peptide of single point-mutated, oncogenic ras proteins. J Exp Med 173:273–276
10. Gedde-Dahl III T, Eriksen JA, Thorsby E, Gaudernack G (1992) T cell responses against products of oncogenes. Generation and characterization of human T cell clones specific for p21 ras derived synthetic peptides. Hum Immunol 33:266–274
11. Gedde-Dahl III T, Spurkland A, Eriksen JA, Thorsby E, Gaudernack G (1992) Memory T cells from a patient with follicular thyroid carcinoma recognize peptides derived from mutated p21 ras (61 Gln→Leu). Int Immunol 4:1331–1337
12. Gedde-Dahl III T, Fossum B, Eriksen JA, Thorsby E, Gaudernack G (1993) T cell clones specific for p21 ras derived peptides: characterization of their fine specificity and HLA restriction. Eur J Immunol 23:754–760
13. Fossum B, Gedde-Dahl III T, Hansen T, Eriksen JA, Thorsby E, Gaudernack G (1993) Overlapping epitopes encompassing a point mutation (12 Gly→Arg) in p21 ras can be recognized by HLA-DR, -DP and -DQ restricted T cells. Eur J Immunol 23:2687–2691
14. Gedde-Dahl III T, Eriksen JA, Thorsby E, Gaudernack G (1993) In: Lemoine N, Epenetos A (eds) Mutant Oncogenes. Targets for Therapy. Chapman and Hall Medical, London, pp 99–105
15. Fossum B, Gedde-Dahl III T, Breivik J, Eriksen JA, Spurkland A, Thorsby E, Gaudernack G (1994) p21-ras peptide-specific T-cell responses in a patient with colorectal cancer. $CD4^+$ and $CD8^+$ T cells recognize a peptide corresponding to a common mutation (13Gly→Asp). Int J Cancer 56:40–45
16. Fossum B, Breivik J, Meling GI, Gedde-Dahl III T, Hansen T, Knutsen I, Rognum TO, Thorsby E, Gaudernack G (1994) A K-ras 13Gly→Asp mutation is recognized by HLA-DQ7 restricted T cells in a patient with colorectal cancer. Modifying effect of DQ7 on established cancers harbouring this mutation? Int J Cancer 58: 506–511
17. Gedde-Dahl III T, Spurkland A, Fossum B, Wittinghofer A, Thorsby E, Gaudernack G (1994) T cell epitopes encompassing the mutational hotspot position 61 of p21 ras. Promiscuity in ras peptide binding to HLA. Eur J Immunol 24: 401–414
18. Peace DJ, Chen W, Nelson H, Cheever MA (1991) T cell recognition of transforming proteins encoded by mutated ras proto-oncogenes. J Immunol 146: 2059–2065
19. Tsang KY, Nieroda CA, De Filippi R, Chung YK, Yamaue H, Greiner JW, Schlom J (1994) Induction of human cytotoxic T cells lines directed against point-mutated p21 ras-derived synthetic peptides. Vaccine Res 3:183–193
20. Ngo-Giang-Huong N, Kayibanda M, Deprez B, Levy J-P, Guillet J-G, Tilkin A-F (1995) Mutations in position 61 of H-ras p21 protein influence MHC class II presentation. Internat Immunol 7:269–275
21. Johansen BH, Gedde-Dahl III T, Sollid LM, Vartdal F, Thorsby E, Gaudernack G (1994) Binding of ras oncogene peptides to purified HLA-DQ6 (alpha 1*0102, beta 1*0602) molecules. Scand J Immunol 39:607–612

22. Quin H, Chen W, Takahashi M, Disis ML, Byrd DR, McCahill L, Bertram KA, Fenton RG, Peace DJ, Cheever MA (1995) $CD4^+$ T-cell immunity to mutated ras proteins in pancreatic and colon cancer patients. Cancer Res 55:2984–2987
23. Peace DJ, Smith JW, Disis ML, Chen W, Cheever MA (1993) Induction of T cells specific for the mutated segment of oncogenic p21 ras protein by immunization in vivo with the oncogenic protein. J Immunother 14:110–114
24. Yin L, Lowe P, Stauss HJ (1993) T cell recognition of a point mutation in the p21 ras protein. Leukemia 7:27–30
25. Fenton RG, Taub DD, Kwak LW, Smith MR, Longo DL (1993) Cytotoxic T-cell response and in vivo protection against tumor cells harbouring activated ras proto-oncogenes. J Natl Cancer Inst 85:1294–1302
26. Skipper J, Stauss HJ (1993) Identification of two cytotoxic T lymphocyte-recognized epitopes in the ras protein. J Exp Med 177:1493–1498
27. Peace DJ, Smith JW, Chen W, You S-G, Cosand WL, Blake J, Cheever MA (1994) Lysis of ras-oncogene transformed cells by specific cytotoxic T lymphocytes elicited by primary in vitro immunization with mutated ras peptide. J Exp Med 179: 473–479
28. Abrams SL Stanziale SF, Lunin SD, Zaremba S, Sclom J (1996) Identification of overlapping epitopes in mutant ras oncogene peptides that activate $CD4^+$ and $CD8^+$ T cell responses. Eur J Immunol 26:435–443
29. Chicz RM, Urban RG, Gorga JC, Vagnali DAA, Lane WS, Strominger JL (1993) Specificity and promiscuity among naturally processed peptides bound to HLA-DR alleles. J Exp Med 178:27–47
30. Fossum B, Olsen AC, Thorsby E, Gaudernack G (1995) $CD8^+$ T cells from a patient with colon carcinoma, specific for a p21-RAS derived peptide (13GLY→ASP) are cytotoxic towards a carcinoma cell line harbouring the same mutation. Cancer Immunol Immunother 40:165–172
31. van Elsas A, Nijman HW, van der Minne CE, Mourer JS, Kast WM, Melief CJM, Schrier P (1995) Induction and characterization of cytotoxic T-lymphocytes recognizing a mutated p21 ras peptide presented by HLA-A*0201. Int J Cancer 61: 389–396
32. Rammensee H-G, Friede T, Stevanovic S (1995) MHC motifs and peptide ligands: First listing. Immunogenetics 41:178–228
33. Mukherji B, Chakraborty NG, Yamasaki S, Okino T, Yamase H, Sporn JR, Kurzman SK, Ergin MT, Ozols J, Meehan J, Mauri F (1995) Induction of antigen-specific cytolytic T cells in situ in human melanoma by immunization with syngeneic peptide-pulsed autologous antigen presenting cells. Proc Natl Acad Sci USA 92:8078–8082

Idiotype-Based Immunotherapy of Cancers

S. V. Kaveri and M. D. Kazatchkine

Introduction

Idiotypes are sets of antigenic determinants (idiotopes) expressed by variable (V) regions of immunoglobulin molecules (Kunkel et al. 1963; Oudin and Michel 1963). The terminology often extends to antigenic determinants of V regions of T cell receptors. Thus, each antibody molecule, B cell clone, and T cell clone possess unique idiotypes that characterize the structural diversity of V regions of T and B cell clones. Idiotopes are defined serologically by their complementary anti-idiotypic antibodies. Thus, idiotypes, per se, are not physicochemical entities, even though they have a structural basis that is largely or entirely within the hypervariable regions or complementarity-determining regions (CDRs) of the immunoglobulin variable domain. The hypervariable sequences that provide the structural basis for idiotypic determinants reflect inherited germline diversity in the case of natural, unmutated antibodies, and somatic mutations of V genes in the case of antigen-driven antibody responses. An idiotype that is encoded by germ line V genes may be shared by several antibody molecules that recognize an antigen (cross-reactive idiotype, CRI), whereas idiotopes that arise from somatic events define the products of only one or a few clones of antibody-producing B cells (private idiotype) (Kohler et al. 1988).

Idiotypes are relevant for immunoregulation because they are immunogenic (Jerne 1974). Thus, immune responses can be induced in an individual against self-idiotopes of immunoglobulins and of antigen receptors expressed by lymphocytes of that individual. The antibody directed against a nominal antigen (Ab1) interacts via its paratope with the antigen. Within the idiotypic network, Ab1 also reacts through the paratope with an idiotope expressed by a complementary antibody (Ab2) or acts as an antigen when its idiotope is bound by the paratope of a complementary immunoglobulin molecule. In either case, clonal expansion of anti-idiotypic B cells bearing Ab2 immunoglobulin molecules that bind or are bound by the Ab1 will occur. Ab2 anti-idiotypes may be used for targeted immunoregulation. Thus, for example, if an autoimmune disease is secondary to an oligoclonal population of pathogenic Ab1 autoantibodies that carry a specific idiotype, specific suppression of Ab1 antibodies may be achieved by different experimental means with complementary anti-idiotypes (Pawlak et al. 1973). Ab2 anti-

Symposium in Immunology VI
Eibl/Huber/Peter/Wahn (Eds.)

idiotypes specific for the paratope of an Ab1 antibody can influence immune responses only against that antigen, a concept that is essential for immune regulation with anti-idiotype-based therapies. Such anti-idiotypes are referred to as Ab2β antibodies.

Within the population of Ab2β anti-idiotypes, there are antibodies that mimic the nominal antigen, termed "internal images" of the antigen. The concept of internal image is central to the network theory. In Jerne's concept of the idiotypic network, each idiotope expressed by a V region is similar to an epitope of one or several antigens (Jerne 1974). Internal images thus represent the common antigenic determinants between idiotopes on immunoglobulins and cells of the individual and epitopes (antigens) of the outside world. The validity of the concept of the internal image has been established in several experimental systems where, for example, a subset of Ab2β antibodies raised against an Ab1 directed towards a hormone, has been shown to act in an agonistic fashion to the hormone (the nominal antigen for the Ab1) in stimulating hormone-receptor-expressing target cells (Guillet et al. 1985; Sege and Peterson 1978). Mimicry of the nominal antigen by Ab2β antibodies carrying the internal image of the antigen has been used to elicit Ab3 anti-anti-idiotypic antibodies that would resemble Ab1 and express its functional properties upon reaction with the nominal antigen (Kohler et al. 1989). As discussed later in this review, idiotypic "vaccination" using appropriate Ab2β antibodies as immunogens has proven to be a promising approach in active immunotherapy of tumors. Anti-idiotypes that bind to antigenic determinants on V regions that are close to the paratope and sterically inhibit the antigen-Ab1 interaction without being an internal image of the nominal antigen, have been termed Ab2γ antibodies (Bona et al. 1986).

Anti-idiotypes that bind to antigenic determinants on V regions that are close to but not within the paratope and do not inhibit the antigen–Ab1 interaction are referred to as Ab2α. Ab2α antibodies may exert broad regulatory functions as they may react with Ab1 antibodies expressing different paratopic specificities; in other terms, similar α idiotopes may be present on immunoglobulin molecules of different specificities. Anti-idiotypic antibodies against α determinants may be primarily induced by an Ab1 antibody that is specific for one antigen but may bind to immunoglobulins specific for other antigens and therefore regulate immune responses against multiple antigens.

The concepts that were developed with idiotypes of immunoglobulins may equally apply to variable regions of antigen receptors on T lymphocytes. Idiotypes may stimulate the production of antibodies and T cells specific for idiotypic determinants. Therefore responses elicited by immunization with idiotypes or anti-idiotypes can be both humoral and cell-mediated.

Targeted idiotype-based immunointervention utilizes different approaches. Passive immunotherapy takes advantage of, e.g., specific anti-tumor activity of anti-idiotypic antibodies prepared against patients' tumor-specific idiotypic determinants of lymphoma cells or a shared idiotype restricted to a specific tumoral tissue. Active immunotherapy and idiotypic vaccination use anti-idiotypic antibody directed against idiotypes of antibodies which bear the internal image of a nominal antigen as an immunogen. Internal image anti-idiotypes mimic the three dimensional shapes of antigens and thus are effective across the species barrier and are not genetically restricted. The vaccine potential lies in the fact that the Ab2βs would stimulate an antigen-specific immune response.

Idiotype-based vaccines do not contain nominal antigen and hence are economical to produce; in addition they are free from the hazards of transmitting contaminating infectious agents. As the idiotype vaccines are proteins in nature, they can be conjugated to carrier molecules to render the antigens T-cell dependent, thus receiving maximum T-cell help. From earlier studies, it is clear that T-cell-dependent antigen evokes a better immune response than a T-cell-independent antigen. Synthetic idiotype vaccines may be envisaged as it is possible to design peptides that represent the relevant idiotypic structures necessary to induce the desired vaccination effect. It has been shown that an acquired tolerance to a given antigen may be abolished by using a different molecular form of the same antigenic moiety. This has particular relevance as far as immunotherapy in cancer patients is concerned. The validity of passive and active anti-idiotypic therapy has been successfully demonstrated in tumoral, bacterial, viral, and parasitic models (Bhattacharya-Chatterjee et al. 1994).

Idiotype-Based Immunotherapy of Cancers

Tumor cells are recognized as foreign and elicit specific humoral and cellular immune responses. Antitumor immunity may be associated with the spontaneous regression of tumors in patients, providing a conceptual basis for active immunotherapy of cancer. Anti-idiotypic antibodies bearing internal images of tumor antigens are candidates of choice in the strategy of tumor immunotherapy. A large number of experimental studies have validated this approach (Bhattacharya-Chatterjee et al. 1994).

The identification of tumor-specific antigens that would distinguish between a malignant and a normal cell is relevant for tumor diagnosis, prophylaxis and therapy. However, the existence of tumor-specific antigens remains unproven in the majority of human cancers. The following are some of the antigens that meet most criteria to be targets for specific immunotherapy. The gp37 antigen is a well-characterized glycoprotein antigen associated with acute lymphoblastic leukemia and cutaneous T-cell lymphoma that is not expressed on normal T cells. The carcinoembryonic antigen (CEA), a 180 kDa glycoprotein, is expressed in a broad spectrum of human tumors and has been used to monitor tumor progression. Some of the anti-CEA antibodies that have been generated react with an epitope that is specific for the glycoprotein, whereas others react with antigens present in normal human tissue. Melanoma-associated chondroitin-sulfate proteoglycan is expressed on the majority of melanoma tumor cells and to some extent on keratinocytes and endothelial cells. High molecular weight melanoma-associated antigen (HMW-MAA) is expressed with high density on a large percentage of melanoma lesions with limited heterogeneity and has restricted distibution in normal tissues. A selected number of studies that are relevant for the treatment of human tumors are discussed here.

Immunotherapy of B-cell Lymphomas

The idiotype expressed by the V regions of surface immunoglobulins represents a distinct marker of B lymphoma cells and thus a potential target for therapeutic intervention with anti-idiotype antibody. Surface immunoglobulin would be Ab1 and the Ab2s raised against the Ab1 would be used for treatment.

An initial trial used polyclonal goat anti-idiotype against surface immunoglobulin in a patient with lymphocytic leukemia. Administration of the antibody resulted in a decrease in the number of circulating leukemic cells but was associated with serious side effects (Hamblin et al. 1980). Miller and Levy have carried out a series of trials using custom-made mouse monoclonal anti-idiotypic antibodies specific for idiotypes of surface immunoglobulins of B-cell lymphomas. Their first trial involved a patient who was treated with 150 mg of an anti-idiotypic antibody which reacted exclusively with the patient's B cells (Miller et al. 1982). The patient was repeatedly infused in order to reduce the level of circulating idiotype. The immunoglobulins expressing the idiotype disappeared and a reduction in the volume of the tumor occurred. Several parameters including volume of liver, number of platelets, and hemoglobin levels returned to normal. Direct binding of anti-idiotype antibody to the surface of malignant cells from lymph nodes was demonstrated. Treatment with anti-idiotype was followed by remission which persisted beyond the half-life of infused antibodies. Possible mechanisms of antibody-mediated killing of tumor cells may include complement-dependent lysis, antibody-dependent cellular cytotoxicity, and phagocytosis of antibody-coated cells by the reticuloendothelial system. A role for hemolytic complement is unlikely because of the difficulty in demonstrating lytic effects of mouse antibodies on human cells in vitro using homologous complement. Indirect mechanisms could involve the triggering of an active antitumor response by the anti-idiotype antibody which could outlast the direct effects of the administered anti-idiotypic antibody. It has also been suggested that anti-idiotypic antibodies may induce tumor regression via a direct apoptotic effect on the tumor cells. Vuist et al. (1994) have found a correlation between the ability of an anti-idiotypic antibody to induce an increase in tyrosine phosphorylation in vitro and its ability to induce tumor regression in the patient. It has also been suggested that antibodies to growth signalling receptors may act as agonists which induce the arrest of cellular proliferation and lead to a transient state of tumor dormancy. As most remissions induced by anti-idiotypic antibodies are eventually followed by lymphoma relapse, it may be that growth-arrest signals mediated by the interaction of the anti-idiotype antibody with surface immunoglobulin is involved in the induction of a dormancy state that is terminated due to the emergence of a resistant lymphoma cell variant (Yefenof et al. 1993) or to the failure of low-grade immunity stimulated by the dormant tumor cells (Dyke et al. 1991),

Further attempts at passive therapy of B-cell lymphomas were less successful. In a trial carried out with ten patients, five patients showed secondary reactions and five others showed partial and transient recovery (Meeker et al. 1985a). The decreased efficacy of anti-idiotype antibody therapy in B-cell neoplasms may be due to modulation of the antibody at the cell surface, failure to elicit effective cytotoxicity despite antibody binding, or the occurrence of multiple clones in a single patient. In addition, a neoplasm can escape anti-idiotype antibody detection through the emergence of a subclone which, although derived from the parent neoplasm and similar in all respects to it, expresses an altered idiotype. This alteration renders the immunoglobulin inaccessible to therapeutic anti-idiotype antibody. Such a phenomenon has been observed in one patient in whom the spontaneous change of idiotype became evident during regrowth of the lymphoma shortly after an abrupt tumor regression (Raffeld et al. 1985). In this particular patient, analysis of V regions indicated no change in V gene rearrangement but rather a somatic mutation of the V region. In two patients, changes in the expression of the idiotype were associated with a switch from μ to γ heavy chain expression (Meeker et al. 1985b). In addition, patients with B-cell lymphoma may have a tumor cell population that fails to react with an anti-idiotypic antibody because of the coexistence within the tumor of two totally separate clones of neoplastic B-cells (biclonal lymphoma; Sklar et al. 1984).

The effect of anti-idiotype antibody therapy has also been evaluated in combination with either interferon-α (IFN-α) or chlorambucil (Brown et al. 1989; Maloney et al 1992). Anti-idiotype antibody therapy in combination with IFN-α resulted in complete tumor regression that lasted for over 5 years with no further therapy in three of 11 patients. In the trial in which the anti-idiotype antibody was administered in combination with chlorambucil (13 patients), one patient underwent a complete remission, eight had a partial remission and two exhibited minor remission, suggesting that inclusion of a chemotherapeutic agent does not prevent the emergence of idiotype-negative tumor cells. Although custom-made monoclonal anti-idiotype antibody therapy is promising in patients having failed chemotherapy, the procedure involves identification and characterization of the tumor-associated idiotype and fusion and screening of hybridomas which is time-consuming and labor intensive and requires viable tumor cells for screening. Identification of shared idiotopes on tumor cells from multiple patients has provided an advantage in designing therapeutic monoclonal anti-idiotypic antibodies (Miller et al. 1989).

In order to overcome the drawback of poor immunogenicity of V regions of immunoglobulins expressed on malignant B cells and to avoid the use of potentially toxic immunological adjuvants, idiotype/granulocyte-macrophage colony-stimulating factor fusion proteins have been recently developed as vaccines for B-cell lymphomas (Tao and Levy 1993). Yet another approach to improve the idiotype-based immunotherapy is the application of bispecific antibody technology which allows targeting of T cells by using bispecific IgG that links the T-cell receptor complex to a tumor-associated antigen, resulting in T cell-mediated lysis of tumor targets (Demanet et al. 1992; Weiner and Hillstrom 1991).

Immunotherapy of Acute Lymphoblastic Leukemia and Cutaneous T-cell Lymphoma

Preliminary approaches in this area have used active immunotherapy based on the preparation of Ab2s bearing internal images of tumor antigens. Anti-idiotypic antibodies have been prepared against a monoclonal antibody which recognizes the tumor-specific gp37 antigen. Four patients were treated with first dose level (1 mg/intradermal injection) of alum-precipitated murine IgG1 monoclonal anti-idiotypic antibody 4DC6 (Bhattacharya-Chatterjee et al. 1994). One patient was treated intradermally three times every 2 weeks. Whereas pretreatment serum was almost negative for human anti-mouse antibodies (HAMAs), a significant HAMA response was induced following the second immunization with 4DC6. A major portion of the HAMA was directed against the idiotype of 4DC6. The anti-anti-idiotype (Ab3) response increased after the third immunization and reached a plateau thereafter. Although binding of radiolabeled Ab1 to Ab2 was inhibited by more than 50 % by the patient's serum, the binding of labeled Ab1 to gp37-positive MOLT-4 cells was inhibited by less than 15 %, indicating that only a minor fraction of the Ab3 was tumor specific.

Another patient presented with a T cell lymphoma of intermediate grade confined to the skin with large masses in the neck, arms, shoulders, and trunk. A clinical response was noted following the second immunization with 4DC6 and was associated with a delayed-type hypersensitivity reaction at the injection site. With each ensuing injection, the patient's Ab3 titer kept increasing. In addition, lymphocytes isolated from patient's blood showed anti-idiotype-specific cellular immunity as assessed by a T-cell proliferation assay. The patient's recovery lasted for several months, with more than 90 %

regression of tumor masses. There was no clinical improvement in one patient following several immunizations, and one patient did not mount a HAMA response. Toxicity in the four patients was negligible.

Immunotherapy of Colorectal and Pancreatic Cancers

Goat polyclonal anti-idiotypic antibodies that functionally mimic the antigens defined by the anti-colorectal carcinoma antibodies 17-1A and GA 733 were generated. The antibodies emulsified in alum were injected intradermally into 30 patients with colorectal cancer (Herlyn et al., 1987). All patients developed Ab3 that bound to and competed with Ab1 for binding to colorectal tumor cells. Ab3 antibodies could be eluted from tumor cells and shown to bind to purified antigen. There was regression of tumor in six patients and stabilization of the condition in seven. The disease progressed in 17 patients despite the treatment. No side effects were observed. In a follow-up trial (Herlyn et al. 1991), a different goat polyclonal Ab2 was administered to 12 patients who had previously been diagnosed with colorectal carcinoma but whose tumors were excised prior to Ab2 therapy. Of the six patients who developed tumor-specific Ab3, two also exhibited antigen-specific T cells which proliferated in culture upon stimulation with GA 733. Of the 12 patients, seven showed tumor regression which lasted between 1 and 4 years following treatment.

A recent phase I trial has used a human monoclonal Ab2 that interacts with the binding site of Ab1 directed against the gp 72 antigen in patients with advanced colorectal carcinoma (Robins et al. 1991). Proliferative responses to gp-72-positive tumor cells were observed in four of five patients tested that correlated with responses to Ab2 in most of the patients. No toxicity related to anti-idiotype immunization was seen. The potential therapeutic implication of the idiotypic cascade has further been demonstrated in patients with advanced adenocarcinoma of the pancreas treated with a single infusion of Ab1 together with autologous leukocytes (Wettendorf et al. 1989). The ability of the patients to produce Ab3 that bound to autologous Ab2s was shown using culture supernatants of peripheral blood mononuclear cells from Ab1-treated patients following stimulation of the cells with heterologous Ab2 that functionally mimicked the tumor antigen defined by Ab1. Ab3 shared idiotopes with Ab1 and was Ab1-like in its binding specificity to tumor cells, antigen, and Ab2.

The importance of anti-idiotype-reactive T cells for antitumor responses in immunotherapy using mAbs has been studied by Fagerberg et al. (1994). Induction of Ab2 and Ab3 as well as of the corresponding T cells (T2 and T3) was evaluated following treatment with an Ab1 in patients with colorectal carcinoma. All patients developed Ab2 and Ab3 with Ab1-like properties whereas only half of the patients developed Ab3-like T cells. Patients with anti-idiotype-specific T cells showed tumor reduction following therapy whereas patients lacking a detectable T-cell response failed to respond to treatment. The same group further demonstrated that human anti-idiotypic antibodies are capable of inducing a humoral and cellular immune response against a colorectal carcinoma-associated antigen (Fagerberg et al. 1995).

Immunotherapy of Melanoma

Extensive work has been carried out in patients with melanoma with promising results. The development of monoclonal antibodies against a membrane-bound melanoma-associated antigen referred to as HMW-MAA has allowed the design of several trials of active specific immunotherapy. HMW-MAA represents a useful target for active and passive immunotherapy because of its high density and frequency on melanoma lesions, limited heterogeneity, and restricted distribution in normal tissues.

In the first trial, an anti-idiotype antibody against an idiotope within the antigen-combining site of a syngeneic anti-HMW-MAA antibody 225.28 was used (Mittelman et al. 1990). The anti-idiotype antibody MF11-30, which bears the internal image of HMW-MAA, was administered subcutaneously to seven patients with stage IV malignant melanoma in a phase I trial. The lowest and highest cumulative dose of immunizing anti-idiotype MF11-30 was 1.5 and 17.5 mg respectively, with an average of 9.5 mg per patient. The average time of treatment was 43 weeks. None of the immunizations were associated with toxicity although HAMAs were detected. Minor clinical responses which lasted for 34–83 weeks were observed in three patients with a decrease in pulmonary, testicular, and/or cutaneous lesions.

In the second trial, the anti-idiotype antibody was administered to 21 patients at a dose of 2 mg per injection. In 17 of 19 patients, there was an increase in HAMA and 16 developed antibodies that inhibited the interaction of Ab1 and Ab2. One patient achieved a complete remission for a duration of 95 weeks. Minor responses were observed in three patients.

In the third trial, 25 patients with stage IV melanoma were immunized subcutaneously with 2 mg of the mouse monoclonal anti-idiotype antibody MK2-23 which bears the internal image of HMW-MAA defined by Ab1 763.74 (Mittelman et al. 1992). Patients were immunized with the anti-idiotype antibody conjugated with keyhole limpet hemocyonin (KLH) and mixed with BCG. Only 14 of 25 patients developed HAMAs. Ab3 antibodies were found in four patients. Among the patients who developed anti-HMW-MAA Ab3 antibodies, three patients achieved partial remission. The reponses lasted between 52 and 93 weeks. The survival of patients who developed anti-HMW-MAA antibodies was significantly longer than that of patients who had not developed the antibodies. By analyzing the anti-HMW-MAA antibody response in mice at monoclonal level, Kageshita and coworkers dissected the fine specificity and idiotypic profile of the Ab3 population (Yang et al. 1993). This information should be of use in understanding the structural basis for the HMW-MAA antibody response and improving therapeutic strategies.

References

Bhattacharya-Chatterjee M, Foon KA, Kohler H (1994) Idiotypic antibody immunotherapy of cancer. Cancer Immunol Immunotherap 38:75–82

Bona CA, Kang CY, Kohler H, Monestier M (1986) Epibody: the image of the network created by a single antibody. Immunol Rev 90:115–127

Brown SL, Miller RA, Horning SJ, Czerwinski D, Hart SM, McElderry R, Basham T, Warnke R, Merigan TC, Levy R (1989) Treatment of B cell lymphoma with anti-idiotype antibodies alone and in combination with alpha interferon. Blood 73: 651–657

Demanet C, Brissinck J, Moser M, Leo O, Thielmans K (1992) Bispecific antibody therapy of two murine B-cell lymphomas. Int J Cancer 7:67–68

Dyke RJ, McBride H, George AJT, Hamblin TJ, Stevenson FK (1991) Idiotypic vaccination against B cell lymphoma leads to dormant tumor. Cell Immunol 132:70–83

Fagerberg J, Frodin JE, Ragnahammer P, Steinitz M, Wigzell H, Mellstedt H (1994) Induction of immune network cascade in cancer patients treated with monoclonal antibodies (Ab1). II. Is induction of anti-idiotype-reactive T cells (T3) of importance for tumor response to mAb therapy? Cancer Immunol Immunother 38: 149–159

Fagerberg J, Steinitz M, Wigzell H, Askelof P, Mellstedt H (1995) Human anti-idiotypic antibodies induced a humoral and cellular immune response against a colorectal carcinoma-associated antigen in patients. Proc Natl Acad Sci USA 92: 4773–4777

Guillet JG, Kaveri SV, Durieu O, Delavier C, Hoebeke J, Strosberg AD (1985) β adrenergic agonist activity of a monoclonal anti-idiotypic antibody. Proc Natl Acad Sci USA 82:1781–1785

Hamblin TJ, Abdul-Ahad AK, Gordon J, Stevenson FK, Stevenson GT (1980) Preliminary experience in treating lymphocytic leukemia with antibody to immunoglobulin idiotypes on the cell surface. Br J Cancer 42:495–502

Herlyn D, Wettendorf M, Scmoll E, Iliopoulos D, Schedel I, Driekhausen U, Raab R, Ross AH, Jaksche H, Scriba M, Koprowski H (1987) Anti-idiotype immunization of cancer patients: modulation of the immune response. Proc Natl Acad Sci USA 84: 8055–8059

Herlyn D, Benden A, Kane M, Somasundaram R, Zaloudik J, Sperlagh J, Marks G, Hart E, Ralf C, Wettendorf M, Mastrangelo M (1991) Anti-idiotype cancer vaccines: pre-clinical and clinical studies. In Vivo 5:615–623

Jerne NK (1974) Towards a network theory of the immune system. Ann Inst Pasteur Immunol 125C:373–389

Kohler H, Kieber-Emmons T, Srinivasan S, Kaveri S, Morrow WJW, Muller S, Kang C-Y, Raychaudhuri S (1988) Revised immune network concepts. Clin Immunol Immunopathol 52:104–116

Kohler H, Kaveri S, Kieber-Emmons T, Morrow WJ, Muller S, Raychaudhuri S (1989) Idiotypic networks and nature of molecular mimicry: an overview. Methods Enzymol 178:3–35

Kunkel HG, Mannick M, Williams RC (1963) Individual antigenic specificity of isolated antibodies. Science 140:1218–1219

Maloney DG, Brown SL, Czerwinski D, Liles T, Hart SM, Miller RA, Levy R (1992) Monoclonal anti-idiotype antibody therapy of B cell lymphoma: The addition of a short course of chemotherapy does not interfere with the anti-tumor effect nor prevent the emergence of idiotype-negative variant cells. Blood 80:1502–1510

Meeker T, Lowder J, Maloney DG, Miller RA, Thielemans K, Warnke R, Levy R (1985a) A clinical trial of anti-idiotype therapy for B-cell malignancy. Blood 65: 1349–1363

Meeker T, Lowder J, Cleary ML, Stewart S, Warnke R, Sklar J, Maloney DG, Levy R (1985b) Emergence of idiotype variants during treatment of B-cell lymphoma with anti-idiotype antibodies. N Eng J Med 312:1658–1665

Miller RA, Maloney DG, Warnke R, Levy R (1982) Treatment of B-cell lymphoma with monoclonal anti-idiotype antibody. N Engl J Med 306:517–522

Miller RA, Hart SM, Samoszuk M, Coulter C, Brown SL, Czerwinski D, Kelkenberg J, Royston I, Levy R (1989) Shared idiotypes expressed by human B-cell lymphomas. N Engl J Med 321:851–856

Mittelman A, Chen ZJ, Kageshita T, Yang H, Yamada M, Baskind P, Goldberg N, Puccio C, Ahmed T, Arlin Z, Ferrone S (1990) Active specific immunotherapy in patients with melanoma. J Clin Invest 86:2136–2144

Mittelman A, Chen ZJ, Yang H, Wong GY, Ferrone S (1992) Human high-molecular weight melanoma-associated antigen (HMW-MAA) mimicry by mouse anti-idiotypic monoclonal antibody MK2-23: Induction of humoral anti-HMW-MAA immunity and prolongation of survival in patients with stage IV melanoma. Proc Natl Acad Sci USA 89:466–470

Oudin J, Michel M (1963) Une nouvelle forme d'allotypie des globulines gamma du sérum de lapin apparemment liée à la fonction et à la spécificité anticorps. C R Acad Sci (Paris) 257:805–808

Pawlak LL, Hart DA, Nisonoff A (1973) Requirements for prolonged suppression of an idiotypic specificity in adult mice. J Exp Med 137:1442–1448

Raffeld M, Neckers L, Longo D, Cossman J (1985) Spontaneous alteration of idiotype in a monoclonal B-cell lymphoma: Escape from detection by anti-idiotype. N Engl J Med 312:1653–1658

Robins RA, Denton GWL, Hardcastle JD, Austin EB, Baldwin RW, Durrant LG (1991) Anti-tumor immune response and interleukin-2 production induced in colorectal cancer patients by immunization with human monoclonal anti-idiotypic antibody. Cancer Res 51:5425–5429

Sege K, Peterson PA (1978) Use of anti-idiotypic antibodies as cell-surface receptor probes. Proc Natl Acad Sci USA 75:2443–2447

Sklar J, Cleary ML, Thielmans K, Gralow J, Warnke R, Levy R (1984) Biclonal B-cell lymphoma. N Engl J Med 311:20–27

Tao M, Levy R (1993) Idiotype/granulocyte-macrophage colony-stimulating factor fusion protein as a vaccine for B-cell lymphoma. Nature 362:755–758

Vuist WM, Levy R, Maloney DG (1994) Lymphoma regression induced by monoclonal anti-idiotypic antibodies correlates with their ability to induce Ig signal transduction and is not prevented by tumor expression of high levels of bc1-2 protein. Blood 83:899–906

Weiner GJ, Hillstrom JR (1991) Bispecific anti-idiotype/anti-CD3 antibody therapy of murine B-cell lymphoma. J Immunol 147:4035–4044

Wettendorf M, Iliopoulos D, Tempero M, Kay D, Defrietas E, Koprowski H, Herlyn D (1989) Idiotypic cascades in cancer patients treated with monoclonal antibody Co17-1A. Proc Natl Acad Sci USA 86:3789–3791

Yang H, Chen ZJ, Kageshita T, Yamada M, Ferrone S (1993) Idiotypic cascade in the human high-molecular weight-melanoma-associated antigen system: fine specificity and idiotypic profile of anti-anti-idiotypic monoclonal antibodies. Eur J Immunol 23:1671–1677

Yefenof E, Picker LJ, Scheuermann RH, Vitetta ES, Street NE, Tucker TF, Uhr JW (1993) Induction of B cell tumor dormancy by anti-idiotypic antibodies. Curr Opin Immunol 5:740–744

Heat-Shock-Protein-Based Vaccines against Cancers and Intracellular Infections

P. K. Srivastava

Immunogenicity of Cancers

That inbred rodents can be immunized against their own tumors or against other syngeneic tumors was convincingly demonstrated between 1943 and 1962 (Gross 1943; Prehn and Main 1957; Klein et al. 1960; Old et al. 1962; for a review, see Srivastava and Old 1988). This provided the basis for the idea of immunogenicity of cancers and by deduction, of the existence of tumor-specific antigens. In essence, these studies showed that mice vaccinated with inactivated cancer cells are immune to subsequent challenges of live cancer cells. The phenomenon was shown to be individually tumor-specific, in that mice were immune specifically to the tumors that were used to immunize them and not to other tumors (Basombrio 1970; Globerson and Feldman 1964), hence the nomenclature *individually distinct* tumor rejection antigens.

The demonstration of the immunogenicity of cancer cells led to a search for the cancer-derived molecules which elicit resistance to tumor challenges. The general strategy of these experiments was to fractionate cancer-derived proteins and test them individually for their ability to immunize mice against the cancers from which the fractions were prepared [see Srivastava and Old (1988), Old (1981), and Boon and van der Bruggen (1996) for other approaches to the identification of tumor-specific antigens]. The proteins identified by this method turned out to be related to a class of proteins known as heat shock proteins (HSPs) or stress-induced proteins (Lindquist and Craig 1988). Ironically, instead of being tumor-specific proteins, HSPs are among the most highly conserved and abundant proteins in living systems; they are found across the phylogenetic ladder from archaebacteria to primates and differ only modestly among different species, let alone within an inbred strain. All in all, they are the most unlikely candidates for tumor-specific antigens.

The explanation for the tumor-specific immunogenicity of HSPs lies at the intersection of a number of diverse areas including antigen presentation, protein folding and assembly, and priming of cellular immune response to infection and sheds light on them. Tumor-specific immunogenicity of HSPs also suggests some radically novel opportunities for immunotherapy of human cancers and infectious diseases.

Symposium in Immunology VI
Eibl/Huber/Peter/Wahn (Eds.)

Discovery of Heat Shock Proteins as Tumor-Specific Immunogens against Cancers

A biochemical search for the tumor-derived molecules which elicit tumor-specific protective immunity led to the identification of glycoproteins of 96–110 kDa (gp96) as the active principle in immunization by a number of tumors (Srivastava and Das 1984; Srivastava et al. 1986; Palladino et al. 1987; Udono and Srivastava 1994; Udono et al. 1994; Feldweg and Srivastava 1995; S. Janetzki, N. E. Blachere, M. Daou, and P. K. Srivastava, unpublished). Independently, Ullrich et al. (1986) identified the active immunizing principle from one of the same tumors as 84 and 86 kDa (p84/86) isoforms of one protein. The fortuitous reasons that led to the identification of different proteins from the same tumor are discussed at length elsewhere (Srivastava and Maki 1991). However, sequence characterization of the two molecules revealed that gp96 and p84/86 shared considerable homology (Srivastava et al. 1987, 1988; Maki et al. 1990) and were members of the same HSP family: p84/86 is the cytosolic hsp90 and gp96 is its counterpart in the endoplasmic reticulum (ER), in the same manner as the Grp78 (BiP) is the ER-resident counterpart of the cytosolic hsp70. Gp96 transcripts were subsequently shown to be inducible by heat shock and other stresses (Maki 1991; Altmeyer et al. 1996) and heat shock elements were identified in the 5′ flanking region of the gp96 gene (Maki et al. 1991).

The original observations regarding tumor-specific immunogenicity of HSPs were made with gp96 (Srivastava and Das 1984; Srivastava et al. 1986) and hsp90 (Ullrich et al. 1986). However, recent studies have extended the phenomenon to hsp70 (Udono and Srivastava 1993, 1994).

Immunity elicited by immunization with tumors is tumor-specific: a mouse immunized against a given tumor is resistant to that tumor but not to other tumors (Prehn and Main 1957, Old et al. 1962). This immunity is so exquisitely specific that tumors of the same histological type and induced by the same carcinogen in an inbred colony of mice, or even two tumors induced in the same animal by the same carcinogen, are antigenically distinct (Basombrío 1970; Globerson and Feldman 1964). This phenomenon is not restricted to 3-methylcholanthrene-induced tumors (meth A) but is observed in tumors induced by a wide spectrum of agents including UV-irradiation as well as in spontaneous tumors tested (for review, see Srivastava and Old 1988). The molecular basis of this specificity and diversity has been a continuing enigma in cancer immunology.

In line with the specific immunogenicity of tumors, immunization with HSPs derived from tumors also elicits resistance specific to the tumor from which it is derived, but not to other antigenically distinct tumors. Thus, gp96 isolated from Meth A sarcoma elicits immunity against Meth A but not CMS5. Conversely, CMS5 gp96 immunizes against CMS5 but not Meth A (Srivastava et al. 1986). This specificity has also been observed in immunization with gp96 derived from a rat hepatoma (Srivastava and Das 1984), hsp90 derived from the Meth A sarcoma (Ullrich et al. 1986), and hsp70 obtained from the Meth A sarcoma (Udono and Srivastava 1993).

Like other HSPs, gp96, hsp90, and hsp70 are expressed to varying degrees of abundance in normal tissues as well. However, immunization of mice with gp96 or hsp70 derived from liver or spleen of BALB/c mice does not elicit resistance to Meth A sarcoma (Udono and Srivastava 1993, 1994).

The specificity of immunogenicity of HSPs derived from tumor cells and the lack of tumor-immunogenicity of HSP preparations derived from normal tissues suggested that HSPs might be hot spots for mutations during malignant transformation such that the HSP genes will exhibit variation between normal tissues and tumors and among tumors. However, sequencing of gp96 cDNAs from BALB/c spleen, Meth A and CMS5 did not reveal any tumor-specific, individually distinct polymorphisms (unpublished observations). Moore et al. (1990) also did not find tumor-specific DNA sequence polymorphisms in hsp90 genes. This directed our attention to the role of N-linked sugars of gp96 (there are no O-linked sugars in gp96). However, the following observations ruled out their role in tumor-specific immunogenicity of gp96: (a) Meth A cells cultured in the presence of tunicamycin can be used to specifically immunize BALB/c mice against Meth A; (b) gp96 derived from Meth A cells grown in presence of tunicamycin did not bind to Con A–Sepharose and successfully immunized mice specifically against Meth A (unpublished observations). In the case of hsp90 and hsp70, the question of a role for sugars in the specific immunogenicity does not arise since they are not glycosylated. While it is conceivable that specificity might reside in other posttranslational modifications, it is unlikely in view of the fact that immunity to tumors is T-cell mediated; there is not much precedent for cellular immunity to non-peptide determinants. Thus, there appears little reason to believe that the specific immunogenicity of HSPs lies in HSPs per se.

Hypothesis: HSPs Chaperone Antigenic Peptides

The lack of diversity in HSPs led us to consider molecules associated with them. As the gp96 used to immunize mice is homogeneous by all criteria (a single band on overloaded silver-stained gels; a single amino terminus during Edman degradation; anti-peptide antibody to gp96 depletes a preparation of its immunogenic activity), our attention focused on small moieties. A number of HSPs bind to a wide array of molecules, including peptides (Flynn et al. 1989, 1991), and we proposed that gp96 molecules may not be immunogenic per se, but may act as carriers of antigenic peptides (Srivastava and Maki 1991; Srivastava and Heike 1991). In view of the fact that gp96 is predominantly located in the ER we further suggested that gp96 acts as a peptide-acceptor for peptides transported to the ER and may be accessory to the loading of MHC class I molecules. As hsp70 and hsp90 are cytosolic molecules, we also suggested that these molecules serve to chaperone peptides from the point of their generation (as a result of proteolytic degradation) to the point of their association with TAP molecules in the membrane of the ER. Since this chapter is devoted primarily to vaccination, these ideas will not be dealt with here in detail. For a detailed discussion of those ideas and the evidence for them, the reader is referred to two recent articles (Srivastava et al. 1994; Li and Srivastava 1994).

A key prediction of our hypothesis was that the specific immunogenicity of HSPs should be observed in any antigenic system in which it is tested: if the HSPs chaperone antigenic peptides generated in the cytosol, their immunogenicity should not be restricted to one or a few tumors but should be applicable to all tumors and to all viral and other intracellular antigens. This prediction is now being fulfilled as the number of antigens whose peptides have been shown to be associated with HSPs appears to be practically unlimited. Thus, tumor-specific antigens from chemically induced rat hepatoma (Srivastava and Das 1984), chemically induced BALB/c mouse sarcomas (Srivastava et al. 1986; Ullrich et al. 1986), UV-induced C3H mouse squamous cell carcinoma (S. Janetzki, N. E. Blachere, M. Daou, and P. K. Srivastava, unpublished), spontaneous C57BL/6 mouse lung carcinoma (Y. Tamura and P. K. Srivastava, unpublished), spontaneous C57BL/6 mouse melanoma (Y. Tamura and P. K. Srivastava, unpublished), chemically induced BALB/c mouse colon carcinoma (D. Levey and P. K. Srivastava, unpublished), and nontumor antigens such as defined cytosolic antigens (Arnold et al. 1995), viral antigens (Blachere et al. 1993; Suto and Srivastava 1995; Arnold et al. 1995; Neiland et al. 1996), and minor histocompatibility antigens (Arnold et al. 1995) have been found to be associated with HSPs in at least four independent laboratories. It is the widespread occurrence of this phenomenon that permits extension of the use of HSPs for vaccination against cancers to vaccination against viruses and intracellular bacteria.

Mechanism by which HSP–Peptide Complexes Elicit Specific Immunity

Immunization of mice with gp96 leads to tumor-specific protection that is dependent on CD4+ and CD8+ T lymphocytes (Udono et al. 1994). Similarly, antigen-specific, MHC-class-I-restricted CD8+ cytotoxic T lymphocytes (CTLs) can be generated by immunization with gp96 in a number of systems, as described earlier. The mechanism by which immunization with HSP–peptide complexes elicits a CD8+ response has now begun to become clear. A class-I-restricted response usually requires presentation of antigens through the endogenous pathway, but the HSP–peptide complexes, although provided exogenously, are able to channel the peptides into the class I presentation pathway. A clue into this mechanism emerged from the observation that depletion or functional inactivation of macrophags completely abrogates the tumor-specific immunogenicity of gp96; in contrast, immunization with whole tumor cells is not sensitive to depletion of macrophages (Udono and Srivastava 1994). We proposed that macrophages possess receptors for gp96 and other HSPs, allowing them to bind HSP–peptide complexes which are then directed to the endogenous presentation pathway through a compartment distinct from the lysosomal compartment (Srivastava et al. 1994). We have since demonstrated that the broad outlines of our suggestion are indeed correct: gp96–peptide complexes are taken up by the macrophages (and possibly other professional antigen presenting cells such as bone marrow derived dendritic cells) and the peptides are processed and finally re-presented on the MHC I of the macrophages. These new MHC I–peptide complexes finally stimulate appropriate CTLs. It is likely that part of the reason for the unusual immunogenicity of the HSP–peptide complexes lies in this mechanism: due to the expression by professional antigen presenting cells of costimulatory molecules, MHC–peptide complexes presented by professional antigen presenting cells are far better stimulators of cognate CTLs than fibroblasts or tumor cells. HSP receptors on professional antigen presenting cells are presently being sought and finer details of this pathway are under investigation.

Tumor-Derived HSP–Peptide Complexes as Autologous Patient-Specific, Customized Vaccines

Identification of HSPs as chaperones of antigenic peptides has a direct bearing on immunotherapy of human cancer. One of the major conceptual difficulties in cancer immunotherapy has been the possibility that human cancers, like cancers of experimental animals, are antigenically distinct. Clearly, there is evidence emerging for the existence of common human tumor CTL epitopes (Houghton 1994). Nonetheless, in light of the overwhelming evidence from experimental and human systems, it is reasonable to assume that at the very least, human tumors would show tremendous antigenic diversity and heterogeneity. Therefore, the prospect of identifying the immunogenic antigens of individual tumors from cancer patients (or even "only" several different types of immunogenic antigens if the antigens are shared), is daunting to the extent of being impractical. The observations that HSPs chaperone the entire repertoire of antigenic peptides of the cells from which they are derived circumvent this hurdle and allow, for the first time, a practical method for the generation of customized, patient-specific vaccines against human cancer.

If, however, human tumors turn out to be antigenically cross-reactive and thus fundamentally different from all experimental cancers thus far examined (as outlined in the preceding section), anti-melanoma vaccines could be designed simply on the basis of peptide epitopes of known cross-reactive melanoma antigens instead of HSP–peptide complexes isolated from individual melanomas. It is the premise of this article that HSP–peptide complexes provide a uniquely effective method of vaccination even if the protective antigens of human cancers turn out to be cross-reactive. This premise is elaborated as follows.

First, the antigenic cross-reactivity among human melanomas suggests that once a number of shared melanoma antigens are identified, patients can be immunized with synthetic peptides corresponding to the relevant epitopes and that the vaccinated patients will elicit a CD8+ CTL response. Vaccination with peptides under suitable conditions has indeed been shown to elicit CD8+ CTLs in a number of systems (Noguchi et al. 1994; Schulz et al. 1989). Such conditions usually include the use of incomplete Freund's adjuvant along with large quantities of peptide (~100 μg peptide for a 20-g mouse). This is clearly incompatible with human use. Alternative approaches, such as addition of a lipophilic tail to the peptides have been employed successfully (Schulz et al. 1989) and could be potentially suited for human applications. In this context, vaccination with in vitro reconstituted complexes of human HSPs with the relevant antigenic peptides offers an economical and technologically simple method of vaccination. The ability of HSP–peptide complexes, *administered in saline and without any adjuvants*, to prime naive CD8+ CTLs in vivo has been reported recently (Blachere et al. 1993; Udono et al. 1994). The use of human HSPs and synthetic peptides is also attractive from the point of view of circumventing hazards associated with vaccination of patients with chimeric molecular constructs of unknown toxicity.

Second, vaccination with a given peptide will be effective only for patients with a given HLA allele. If different epitopes from a single molecule are recognized by different HLA alleles (as appears to be the case with tyrosinase; Brichard et al. 1993; Wolfel et al. 1994), a cocktail of peptides will have to be used for vaccination of a general population. Even for a given patient, a cocktail may have to be used, as humans are outbred and possess several restriction elements. A far more effective and simpler alternative will be to isolate HSP–peptide complexes from human cell lines transfected with the relevant gene under the control of a high expression promoter. The HSP–peptide complexes purified from such transfectants will consist of the entire repertoire of antigenic peptides derived from that particular protein. As HSP–peptide binding is proximal to HLA–peptide binding during antigen processing, there is no HLA restriction in the HSP-bound peptides. Peptides capable of binding to all possible HLA alleles will be represented among the HSP–peptide complexes.

Third, the methodology for identifying CTL epitopes of human cancers suggests that these epitopes may represent a significantly biased sample of the antigenic repertoire of human cancers. Generation of cell lines is an essential prerequisite for isolation of CTLs and only a very small proportion of human cancers (less than 2% for breast cancers to about 30% for melanomas) lend themselves to it. Of the tumors from which cell lines are developed, only a small proportion permit the generation of CTLs. Thus, the CTL epitopes identified may represent an atypical and sparse sampling of the cancer antigenic repertoire.

Immunogenicity of cancers represents, in all likelihood, the sum total of immunogenicity of a large number of immunogenic epitopes, and effective anticancer vaccines should include this antigenic multiplicity. HSP–peptide complexes represent such a multicomponent, multivalent vaccine. If cancer antigens are shared and not individually indistinct, the use of HSP–peptide complexes isolated from tumors becomes even simpler, such that these complexes need not be isolated from cancers of individual patients. Instead, they could be purified from a mixture of human melanomas and be used to vaccinate allogeneic melanomas. The lack of HLA-restriction of HSP-bound peptides is a key advantage in this regard. Vaccination with multicomponent, multivalent vaccines rather than single or oligo-component vaccines is also necessary for protection against antigenic escape or preexisting antigenic heterogeneity of human cancers. These considerations indicate that regardless of the cross-reactive or individually distinct nature of human cancer antigens, HSP–peptide complexes offer unique and unprecedented advantages over other existing methods in vaccination against human cancer.

Uniqueness of HSP–Peptide Complexes as Vaccines

The use of HSP–peptide complexes in immunotherapy of human cancer has been discussed in the previous section. This section takes a broader look at the unique and powerful advantages conferred by the HSP–peptide vaccination, not only against cancers but also against viruses and intracellular pathogens. These advantages are as follows:

(a) Knowledge of the antigenic epitopes that elicit immunity is a prerequisite for all forms of vaccination. HSP–peptide-based vaccination circumvents this necessity, as HSPs are naturally complexed with the repertoire of peptides generated in a cell. For this reason it is an ideal means for vaccination against cancers or infections for which the protective epitopes are yet undefined, or where a single epitope may not be sufficient for eliciting immunity. It is also ideal if the infectious agent is so highly variable (in a population-, season-, or individual-specific manner) that the prospect of identifying the immunogenic epitopes for each variant is simply impractical. The application of this point to cancer immunotherapy has been discussed in depth in the previous section.

(b) Even in the case of infectious diseases where the relevant antigenic epitopes have been defined, HSP-based vaccination offers a unique advantage:

HSP–peptide complexes can be readily stripped of their natural peptides and these "empty" HSPs can be reconstituted with known, synthetic peptide epitope(s). The in vitro reconstituted noncovalent HSP–peptide complexes elicit a potent T-cell response to the complexed peptide. Furthermore, if the peptide is conjugated covalently to the HSP, the HSP–peptide complexes elicit potent antibody responses to the complexed peptide (Lussow et al. 1991; Barrios et al. 1992). The application of this point to cancer immunotherapy has been discussed in depth in the previous section.

(c) As HSPs are nonpolymorphic (i.e., they exhibit no allelic diversity, although there are several HSP families), they bind the entire spectrum of peptides regardless of the MHC haplotype of a cell. Thus, a HSP–peptide complex isolated from cells of a given haplotype may be used to vaccinate individuals of other haplotypes (Srivastava et al. 1994; Suto and Srivastava 1995; Arnold et al. 1995).

(d) Vaccination with HSP–peptide complexes elicits CD8+ T cells without the use of live (attenuated or otherwise) agents and in spite of exogenous administration (Blachere et al. 1993; Udono et al. 1994; Suto and Srivastava 1995; Arnold et al. 1995).

(e) HSP–peptide based vaccines are inherently multivalent, or indeed panvalent because HSPs chaperone not one or a few but the entire repertoire of epitopes generated in a cell.

(f) As HSP–peptide complexes can be purified easily to apparent homogeneity, vaccination with such preparations circumvents the risks associated with vaccination with attenuated organisms or undefined biological extracts which contain transforming DNA and immunosuppressive factors such as transforming growth factor-β.

References

Altmeyer A, Maki RG, Feldweg AF, Masur S, Srivastava PK (1996) Cell surface localization of gp96, a KDEL containing heat shock protein of the lumen of the endoplasmic reticulum. Int J Cancer (in press)

Arnold D, Rammensee H-G, Schild HJ (1995) Cross-priming of minor histocompatability antigen specific cytotoxic T lymphocytes upon immunization with heat shock protein gp96. J Exp Med 182:885

Barrios C, Lussow AR, van Embden J, Van der Zee R, Rappuoli R, Costantino P, Louis JA, Lambert, PH, Del Giudice G (1992) Mycobacterial heat shock proteins as carrier molecules II: The use of the 70 kDa mycobacterial heat shock protein as carrier for conjugated vaccines can circumvent the need for adjuvants and BCG priming. Eur J Immunology 22:1365

Basombrío MA (1970) Search for common antigenicities among 25 sarcomas induced by methylchloranthrene. Cancer Res 30:2458–2462

Blachere NE, Udono H, Janetzki S, Li Z, Heike M, Srivastava PK (1993) Heat shock protein vaccines against cancer. J. Immunother 14:352

Boon T, van der Bruggen P (1996) Human tumor antigens recognized by T lymphocytes. J Exp Med 183(3):725
Brichard V, van Pel A, Wolfel T, De Plaen E, Lethe B, Coulie P, Boon T (1993) The tyrosinase gene codes for an antigen recognized by autologous cytolytic T lymphocytes on HLA-A2 melanomas. J Exp Med 178:489
Feldweg AM, Srivastava PK (1995) Cancer research: Molecular heterogeneity of tumor rejection antigen/heat shock protein gp96. Int J Cancer 63:310–314
Flynn GC, Chappell TG, Rothman JE (1989) Peptide binding and release by proteins implicated in the catalysis of protein assembly. Science 245:385–388
Flynn GC, Pohl J, Flocco MT, Rothman JE (1991) Peptide-binding specificity of the molecular chaperone BiP. Nature 353:726–730
Globerson A, Feldman M (1964) Antigenic specificity of benzo(a)pyrene induced sarcomas. J Natl Cancer Inst 32:1229
Gross L (1943) Intradermal immunization of C3H mice against a sarcoma that originated in an animal of the same line. Cancer Res 3:323–326
Houghton AN (1994) Cancer antigens: Immune recognition of self and altered self. J Exp Medicine 180:1–4
Janetzki S, Blachere NE, Srivastava PK (1994) Cognate heat shock protein gp96 preparations from two antigenically distinct UV-induced carcinomas elicit tumor-specific rejection and cytotoxic T lymphocyte response. J Exp Med (submitted)
Klein G, Sjogren HO, Klein E, Hellstrom KE (1960) Demonstration of resistance against methylchloranthrene-induced sarcomas in the primary autochthonous host. Cancer Res 20:1561–1572
Li Z, Srivastava PK (1993) Tumor Rejection Antigen Gp96/Grp94 is an ATPase: Implications for protein folding and antigen presentation. EMBO J 12:3143
Li Z, Srivastava PK (1994) A critical contemplation on the role of heat shock proteins in transfer of antigenic peptides during antigen presentation. In: Rammense H-G, Hammerling G (eds) MHC Molecules: Structural and Functional Aspects. BIM Press 94:37–47
Lindquist S, Craig EA (1988) The heat shock response. Annu Rev Genet 22:631–677
Lussow AR, Barrios C, van Embden J, Van der Zee R, Verdini AS, Pessi A, Louis JA, Lambert PH, Del Giudice G (1991) Mycobacterial heat shock proteins as carrier molecules. Eur J Immunol 21:2297
Maki RG (1991) Ph D Thesis, Cornell University
Maki RG, Old LJ, Srivastava PK (1990) Human Homologue of Murine Tumor Rejection Antigen Gp96: Analysis of Regulatory and Coding regions and Relationship to Stress-Induced Proteins. Proc Natl Acad Sci USA 87:5658–5662
Moore SK, Rijli F, Appella E (1990) DNA and Cell Biology. Gene 56:29–40
Nieland TJF, Tan MCAA, Monnee-van Muijen M, Koning F, Kruisbeek AM, Van Bleek G (1996) Isolation of an immunodominant viral peptide that is endogenously bound to the stress protein gp96/grp94. Proc Natl Acad Sci USA 93:6135–6139
Noguchi YT, Chen YT, Old LJ (1994) A mouse mutant p53 product recognized by CD4+ and CD8+ T cells. Proc Natl Acad Sci USA 91:3171
Old LJ (1981) The Search for Specificity. Cancer Res 41:361–375
Old LJ, Boyse EA, Clarke DA, Carswell EA (1962) Antigenic properties of chemically induced tumors. Ann NY Acad Sci 101:80–106
Palladino MA, Srivastava PK, Oettgen HF, DeLeo AB (1987) Expression of a shared tumor-specific antigen by two chemically induced BALB/c sarcomas. I. Detection by a cloned cytotoxic T cell line. Cancer Res 47:5074–5079
Prehn RT, Main JM (1957) Immunity to methylcholanthrene-induced sacromas. J Natl Cancer Inst 18:769–778

Schulz K, Schild H, Wiesmuller K-H, Jung G, Rammensee H-G (1989) In vivo priming of virus-specific cytotoxic T lymphocytes with synthetic lipopeptide vaccines. Nature 342:561

Srivastava PK (1991) Tumor antigens. Curr Opin Immunol 3:654–658

Srivastava PK, Das MR (1984) Serologically unique surface antigen of a rat hepatoma is also its tumor-associated transplantation antigen. Int J Cancer 33:417–422

Srivastava PK, Heike M (1991) Tumor-specific immunogenicity of stress-induced proteins: Convergence of two evolutionary pathways of antigen presentation. Semin Immunol 3:57–64

Srivastava PK, Maki RG (1991) Stress-induced proteins as tumor antigens. Curr Top Microbiol Immunol 167:109–123

Srivastava PK, Old LJ (1988) Individually distinct transplantation antigens of chemically induced mouse tumors. Immunol Today 9:78–83

Srivastava PK, DeLeo AB, Old LJ (1986) Tumor rejection antigens of chemically induced sarcomas of inbred mice. Proc Natl Acad Sci USA 83:3407–3807

Srivastava PK, Chen Y-T, Old LJ (1987) 5′ Structural analysis of genes encoding polymorphic antigens of chemically induced tumors. Proc Natl Acad Sci USA 84:3807–3811

Srivastava PK, Kozak CA, Old LJ (1988) Chromosomal localization of the gene encoding murine tumor rejection antigen gp96. Immunogenetics 28:205–207

Srivastava PK, Udono H, Blachere NE, Li Z (1994) Heat shock proteins transfer peptides during antigen processing and CTL priming. Immunogenetics 39:93–98

Suto R, Srivastava PK (1995) A mechanism for the specific immunogenicity of heat shock protein-chaperoned peptides. Science 269:1585–1588

Udono H, Srivastava PK (1993) Heat shock protein 70-associated peptides elicit specific cancer immunity. J Exp Med 178:1391

Udono H, Srivastava PK (1994) Relative immunogenicities of Heat Shock Proteins gp96, hsp90 and hsp70 against chemically induced tumors. J Immunol 152:5398–5403

Udono H, Levey DL, Srivastava PK (1994) Cellular requirements for tumor-specific immunity elicited by heat shock proteins: tumor rejection antigen gp96 primes CD8+ T cells in vivo. Proc Natl Acad Sci USA 91:3077–3081

Ullrich SJ, Robinson EA, Law LW, Willingham M, Appella E (1986) A mouse tumor-specific transplantation antigen is a heat-shock related protein. Proc Natl Acad Sci USA 83:3121–3125

Wölfel T, Van Pel A, Brichard V, Schneider J, Seliger B, Meyer zum Büschenfelde K-H, Boon T (1994) Two tyrosinase nonapeptides recognized on HLA A-2 melanomas by autologous CTL. Eur J Immunol 24:759

Subject Index

GPSR Compliance

The European Union's (EU) General Product Safety Regulation (GPSR) is a set of rules that requires consumer products to be safe and our obligations to ensure this.

If you have any concerns about our products, you can contact us on ProductSafety@springernature.com

In case Publisher is established outside the EU, the EU authorized representative is:

Springer Nature Customer Service Center GmbH
Europaplatz 3
69115 Heidelberg, Germany

Batch number: 10704713

Printed by Printforce, the Netherlands